EASY-TO-FOLLOW ANTI-INFLAMMATORY DIET FOR BEGINNERS

QUICK AND SIMPLE MEALS TO REDUCE CHRONIC INFLAMMATION, IMPROVE GUT HEALTH, MANAGE WEIGHT LOSS, AND ENHANCE IMMUNITY

LYNN BENEDETTO

© **Copyright Lynn Benedetto, 2024. All rights reserved.**

The content within this book may not be reproduced, duplicated, or transmitted without direct written permission from the author or publisher.

Under no circumstances will any blame or legal responsibility be held against the publisher or author for any damages, reparations, or monetary losses due to the information contained within this book. You are solely responsible for your own choices, actions, and results, whether they are influenced by the content of this book or not.

Legal Notice:

This book is copyright-protected. This book is only for personal use. You cannot amend, distribute, sell, use, quote, or paraphrase any part of the content within this book without the consent of the author or publisher.

Disclaimer Notice:

Please note that the information contained within this document is for educational and entertainment purposes only. All effort has been expended to present accurate, up-to-date, reliable, and complete information. No warranties of any kind are declared or implied. Readers acknowledge that the author is not engaging in the rendering of legal, financial, medical, or professional advice. The content within this book has been derived from various sources. Please consult a licensed professional before attempting any techniques outlined in this book.

By reading this document, the reader agrees that under no circumstances is the author responsible for any losses, direct or indirect, which are incurred as a result of the use of the information contained within this document, including, but not limited to, — errors, omissions, or inaccuracies.

Medical Disclaimer:

The information provided in this book, Easy-To-Follow Anti-Inflammatory Diet for Beginners: Quick and Simple Meals to Reduce Chronic Inflammation, Improve Gut Health, Manage Weight Loss, and Enhance Immunity, is intended for educational purposes only and is not a substitute for professional medical advice, diagnosis, or treatment. The content is based on research, personal experience, and the author's interpretation of health and nutrition information.

Before starting any new diet, exercise program, or health regimen, it is essential to consult with your healthcare provider or a registered dietitian, especially if you have any pre-existing medical conditions, are pregnant, nursing, or are taking any medications.

The author and publisher of this book are not responsible for any adverse effects or consequences that may result from the use of any suggestions, preparations, or procedures discussed in this book. Individual results may vary, and the success of any dietary changes depends on various factors, including but not limited to genetics, lifestyle, and adherence to the program.

Always seek the advice of a qualified healthcare provider with any questions you may have regarding a medical condition. Never disregard professional medical advice or delay in seeking it because of something you have read in this book.

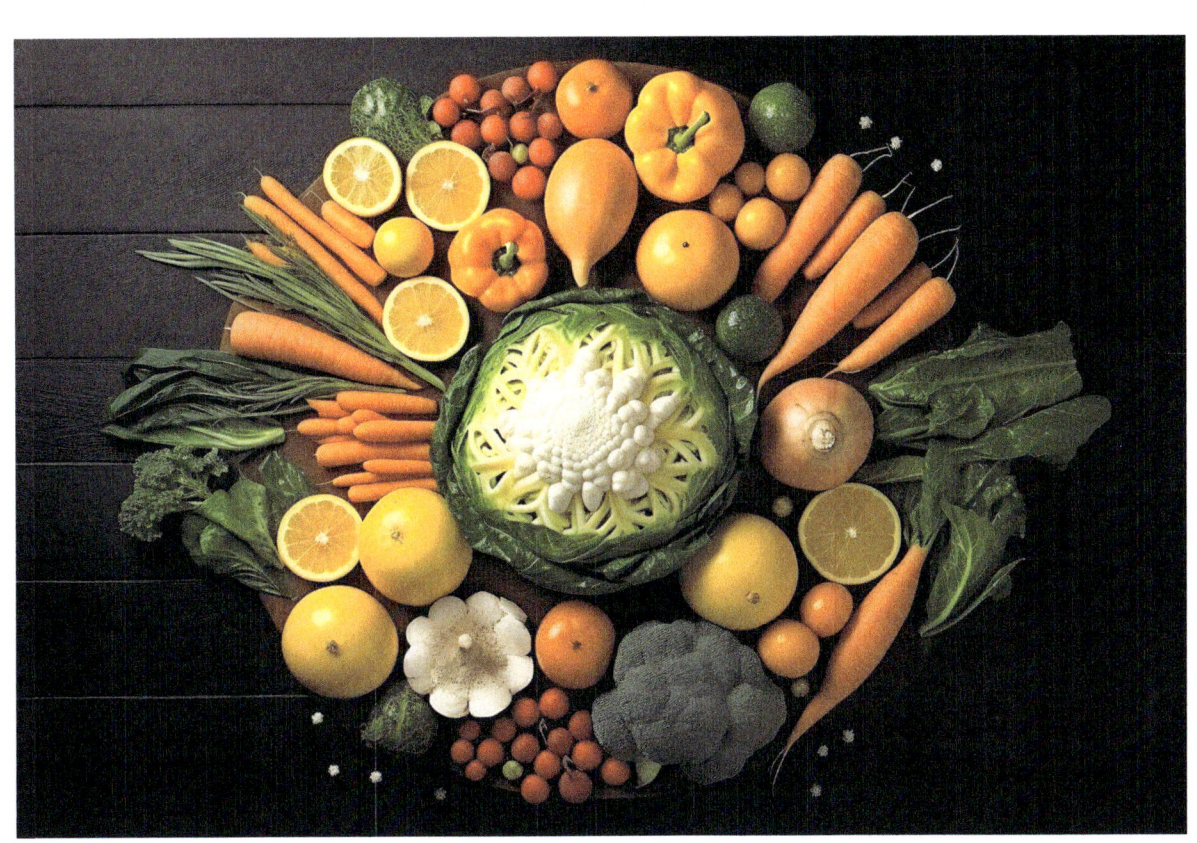

CONTENTS

Introduction 9

1. UNDERSTANDING INFLAMMATION AND ANTI-INFLAMMATORY BASICS 13
   What Is Inflammation? An Overview 13
   Linking Diet and Inflation: Scientific Insights 14
   Essential Anti-Inflammatory Foods to Include in Your Diet 16
   Foods to Avoid: What Triggers Inflammation? 18
   Reading Labels: Identifying Hidden Inflammatory Ingredients 20
   The Anti-Inflammatory Food Pyramid Explained 23

2. SETTING UP FOR SUCCESS ON YOUR DIET JOURNEY 27
   Kitchen Makeover: Preparing Your Space for Success 27
   Budget-Friendly Shopping for Anti-Inflammatory Ingredients 29
   The Art of Meal Prepping: Simple Steps to Save Time 31
   Anti-Inflammatory Cooking Techniques to Maximize Benefits 33
   Managing Dining Out—Making Smart Choices 34
   Addressing Common Diet Transition Challenges 36

3. WEIGHT MANAGEMENT AND NUTRITIONAL INSIGHTS 39
   The Role of an Anti-Inflammatory Diet in Weight Loss 39
   Understanding Calories and Macronutrients in Your Diet 41
   Balancing Carbs, Proteins, and Fats 42
   Nutrient-Dense Foods to Enhance Meal Quality 44
   Tracking Your Progress: Tools and Techniques 46
   Overcoming Weight Loss Plateaus 47

4. SPECIAL DIETARY CONSIDERATIONS AND SUBSTITUTIONS 51
   Gluten-Free Anti-Inflammatory Eating 51
   Dairy Subscriptions in Your Anti-Inflammatory Diet 53
   Vegetarian and Vegan Options for Every Meal 56
   Nut-Free Snacks and Meals for Allergy Sufferers 59
   Low-FODMAP Choices for Sensitive Stomachs 60
   Adapting Recipes for the Whole Family 61

5. ENHANCING GUT HEALTH AND IMMUNITY 67
   The Gut-Health Connection: Basics You Need to Know 67
   Probiotics and Prebiotics: Allies in Your Anti-Inflammatory Diet 69
   Foods That Boost Your Immune System Naturally 71
   Combating Common Digestive Issues with Diet 73
   The Impact of Stress on Gut Health and Immunity 75
   Lifestyle Changes to Support Digestive Health 77

6. **OVERCOMING CHALLENGES AND STAYING MOTIVATED** — 81
   - Dealing with Social and Family Dining Challenges — 81
   - Finding Quick Fixes for Busy Days — 83
   - Handling Cravings and Comfort Food Alternatives — 85
   - Celebrating Success: Rewarding Your Dietary Achievements — 86
   - Building a Support Network: Online and Offline — 87
   - Staying Inspired: Continuously Refreshing Your Meal Plans — 89

7. **SUSTAINING AN ANTI-INFLAMMATORY LIFESTYLE LONG-TERM** — 93
   - Integrating Physical Activity for Comprehensive Benefits — 93
   - Mindfulness and Its Role in Anti-Inflammatory Eating — 96
   - Seasonal Eating: Adjusting Your Diet with the Calendar — 98
   - Advanced Meal Planning: Prepping for Success — 101
   - When to Reassess Your Diet and Make Tweaks — 102
   - Continuing Education: Staying Informed on Nutritional Advances — 104

8. **QUICK AND EASY ANTI-INFLAMMATORY RECIPES** — 107
   - Five-Ingredient Breakfasts to Kickstart Your Day — 107
   - Quick Lunches: Meals in 20 Minutes or Less — 110
   - Simple and Satisfying Anti-Inflammatory Dinners — 112
   - Snacks and Small Bites: Healthy Options on the Go — 115
   - Delicious Smoothies, Juices, Drinks, and Herbal Teas for Inflammation Relief — 116
   - Desserts: Satisfying Your Sweet Tooth the Right Way — 122

Conclusion — 129
References — 131

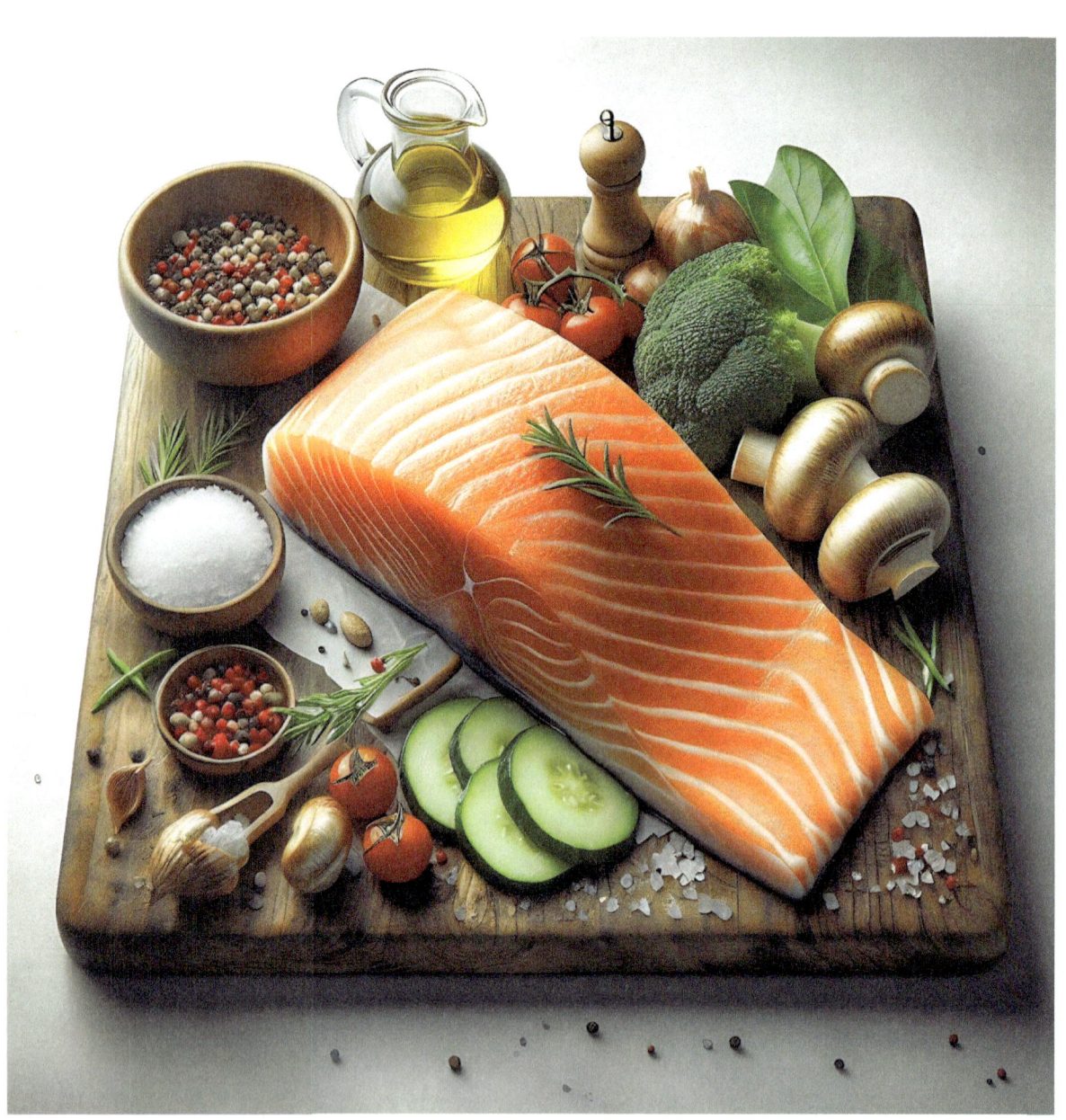

INTRODUCTION

Welcome! If you're picking up this book, it's likely because you're curious about how an anti-inflammatory diet might change your life. I want to reassure you that you're not just starting a diet; you're stepping toward a healthier, more vibrant way of living. It's not just about eating differently; it's about making manageable, informed choices that enhance your overall well-being.

My journey began on an ordinary Tuesday when, after years of dealing with persistent health issues, I stumbled upon an article about the impacts of inflammation on the body—that moment sparked a profound realization: the solution to my discomfort could be as simple as changing what I ate. This insight led me down a path of extensive research and, ultimately, to the creation of this book. I wanted to share what I learned, hoping it could help others as much as it helped me.

This book demystifies the anti-inflammatory diet for beginners. It's filled with straightforward, practical advice grounded in scientific knowledge, aiming to arm you with the tools you need to integrate this diet successfully into your daily life. You'll discover improved gut health and weight management, significant reductions in inflammation-related pain, and a robust boost in your immunity.

What exactly is an anti-inflammatory diet? Simply put, it focuses on whole, nutrient-dense foods and avoids those that trigger inflammatory responses in the body. While this concept is backed by science, we'll keep the explanations light and digestible, saving the deeper dives for your exploration as you grow more confident in your understanding.

The benefits of adopting this way of eating are well-documented and significant. Studies show reductions in chronic pain, enhanced digestive health, and even improvements in mood and energy levels. Each chapter of this book builds on this foundation, from understanding the root causes of inflammation to preparing simple and delicious meals that align with these principles.

The book, structured to be as user-friendly as possible, includes meal plans, shopping guides, and tips on meal preparation. It acknowledges and addresses common challenges like tight schedules, budget constraints, and initial skepticism about the effectiveness of dietary changes. I aim to equip you with the knowledge and practical steps to overcome these hurdles.

As you turn these pages, I encourage you to embrace this learning opportunity with an open mind. Think of this as adopting a new diet and embarking on a healthier life. Remember, the steps you are about to take are the same ones that transformed my health and well-being.

Let's start this journey with the promise that you are not alone. By following the guidance in this book, you can achieve the health goals you set for yourself. Here's to a healthier, happier you!

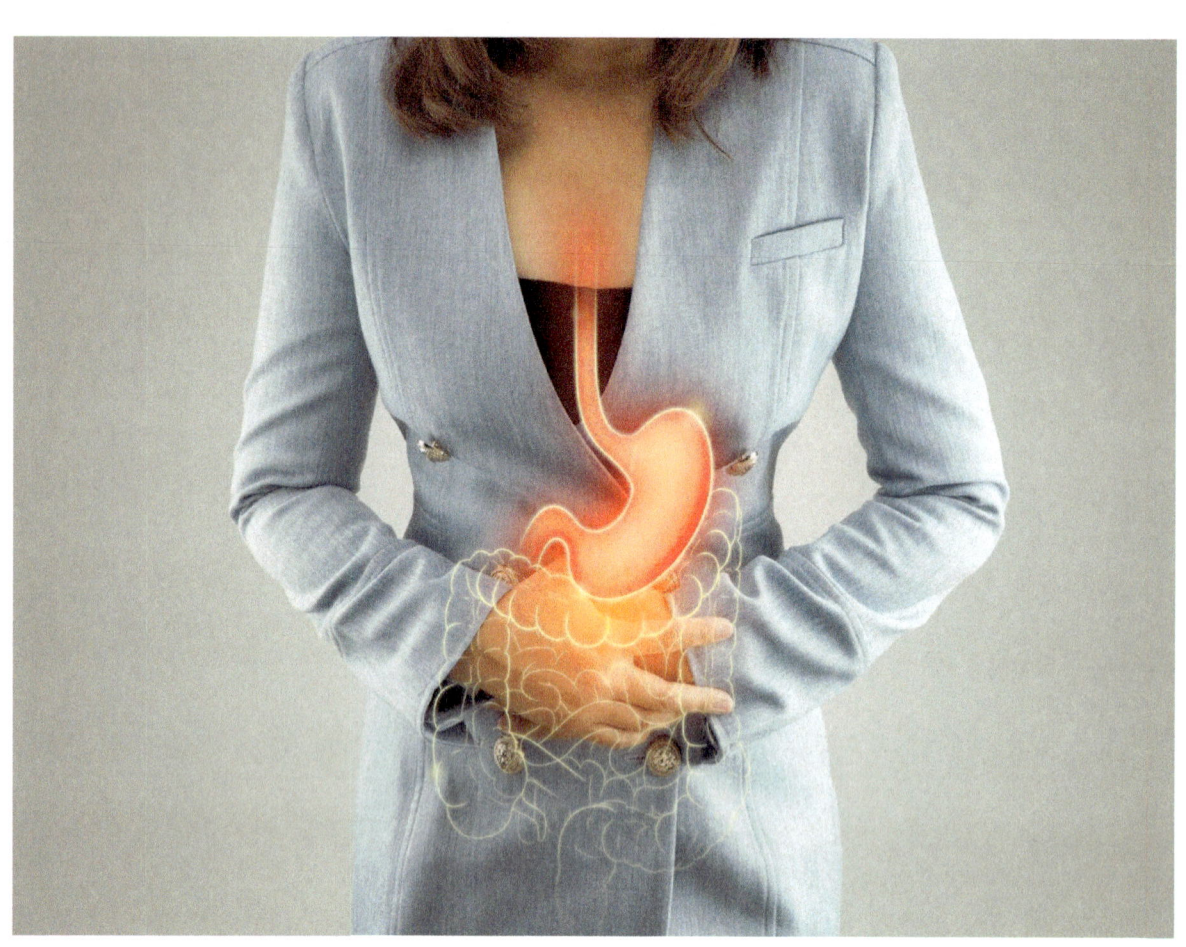

1

UNDERSTANDING INFLAMMATION AND ANTI-INFLAMMATORY BASICS

Did you know that not all inflammation is harmful? Surprising, right? Often, we hear the word "inflammation" and immediately think of unpleasantness—redness, swelling, pain—the classic signs that something might be wrong. However, inflammation is a crucial part of our body's defense mechanism. Our natural alarm system is a biological call to arms against invaders and injuries. But here's the kicker: sometimes, this system can get too overzealous, and that's where problems begin. Like a smoke alarm that goes off every time you make toast, your body's inflammatory response can sometimes overreact to minor irritants or, worse, start seeing parts of your body as a threat. This chapter will walk you through the intricacies of inflammation, define it, outline its benefits, and point out its drawbacks.

WHAT IS INFLAMMATION? AN OVERVIEW

Let us start by clarifying what inflammation is. Picture your body as a well-trained security team, always on guard to protect you. This team takes action when you get a cut, bump, or bruise. In acute inflammation, blood and immune cells rush to the site to treat the issue, causing redness, heat, swelling, and discomfort. It's quick, localized, and crucial injuries wouldn't heal without it. However, imagine that the security team didn't know when to stop, continually fighting long after the initial threat was gone. This scenario describes chronic inflammation, where the inflammatory process persists, leaving your body in a constant state of alertness. This inflammation can lead to numerous long-term health issues, such as arthritis, where joints become inflamed, causing persistent pain and discomfort.

Understanding the biological ballet that occurs during inflammation is fascinating. When cells are damaged, they release substances known as cytokines. Think of cytokines as the flare guns of your cells, signaling distress and calling for backup. These signals trigger your immune system to spring into action, sending white blood cells and other warriors to the scene to fight off invaders, such as bacteria, and begin repairs. This process is essential, but it's all about balance. Too much inflammation, especially where it isn't needed, can be like having too many security guards crowding into a room, getting in each other's way, and potentially causing damage.

The symptoms of inflammation are your body's way of telling you that the security team is doing its job. Redness and heat occur as blood rushes to the site; swelling happens due to fluids accumulating to dilute harmful substances; pain is a signal telling you to take care and not aggravate the injured or infected area further. In cases of chronic inflammation, these symptoms aren't as pronounced as in acute cases and can be misleadingly subtle. That's why chronic inflammation can be particularly treacherous—it plays a long game, and without clear, immediate signs, it can be challenging to know it's happening.

It's essential to recognize that inflammation, by itself, isn't the enemy. It's a natural and critical part of healing. Problems only arise when this response becomes disproportionate or misdirected. That's why understanding inflammation is the first step in taking control of it—knowing when it's helping or harming and how to modify your lifestyle and diet to manage it effectively. This knowledge is powerful; it's the first tool in your toolkit as you learn to fine-tune your body's responses toward a healthier balance.

LINKING DIET AND INFLATION: SCIENTIFIC INSIGHTS

When you think about what you eat daily, it seems like a matter of taste and preference. But did you know that your diet plays a crucial role in managing inflammation within your body? Scientists have been digging into this for years and have uncovered some compelling connections between what we eat and how our bodies manage inflammation. It's not just about avoiding bloating or indigestion after a heavy meal; it's about understanding how certain foods can actively influence inflammation levels in your body, for better or worse.

Let's break it down: Foods aren't just packages of calories and nutrients but signals. They interact with our bodies at a molecular level. Some foods, like those high in processed sugars or unhealthy fats, can trigger an increase in specific inflammatory markers. Think of these foods as being like noisy disruptors in a quiet room. They can cause chaos, leading to an increase in cytokines, which are proteins that promote inflammation. Consuming foods rich in processed sugars or unhealthy fats doesn't just add calories; they actively promote inflammatory processes that can exacerbate conditions like arthritis, heart disease, and even depression.

On the flip side, some foods do the exact opposite. These foods help you reduce inflammation; they are usually high in omega-3 fatty acids, such as walnuts, salmon, and flaxseeds.

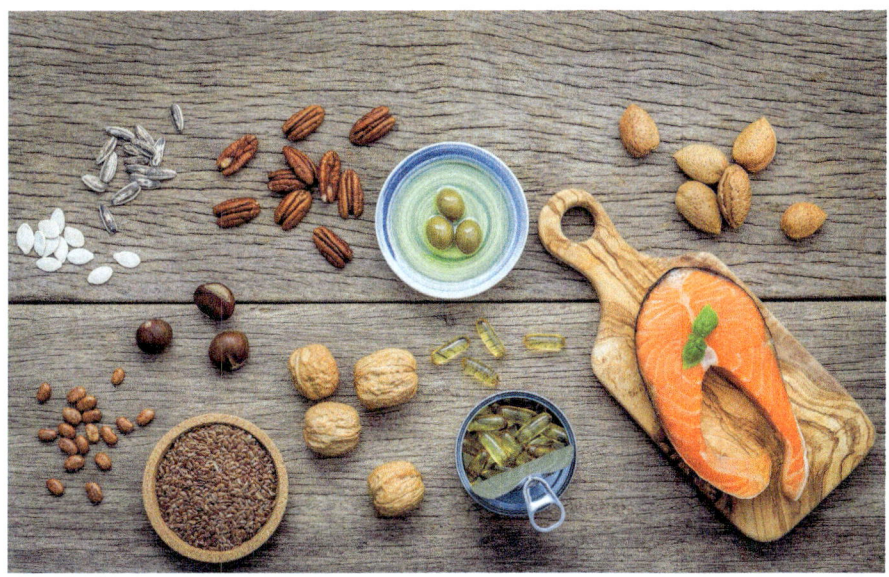

Omega-3 fatty acids are fascinating because they help inhibit the production of inflammatory cytokines. They work at the cellular level to quiet those inflammatory signals, much like turning down the volume on that chaos in the silent room. It's not just omega-3s, though. Many fruits, vegetables, nuts, and whole grains play similar roles. They are abundant in phytochemicals and antioxidants that work to counteract free radicals, which are harmful ingredients that tend to trigger inflammation and oxidative damage

The research on this is robust and growing. For instance, several studies have highlighted that the Mediterranean diet, high in vegetables, fruits, nuts, whole grains, fish, and healthy oils, mainly reduces inflammation. One pivotal study published in the

Journal of the American College of Cardiology found that people following a Mediterranean diet had significantly lower inflammatory markers like C-reactive protein and interleukin-6 levels. Another research piece in the Nutrition & Diabetes journal noted that a diet high in refined starches, sugar, and saturated and trans fats can exacerbate the inflammatory process. In contrast, foods high in omega-3 fatty acids, fiber, and antioxidants can significantly reduce the levels of inflammation.

Understanding the mechanisms by which diet affects inflammation at the molecular level can seem daunting, but it boils down to simple chemistry. Eating anti-inflammatory foods gives your body the tools to manage the repair processes more efficiently and keep the inflammatory response in check. Decreasing the chance of chronic diseases associated with chronic inflammation aids in controlling pain and swelling and offers long-term health advantages.

Thus, our ongoing research on the relationship between nutrition and inflammation reveals that making wise food decisions can be a very effective way to take control of your health. It's not about following a strict diet or denying yourself the foods you love, but understanding the balance and making choices that help support your body's natural defenses against inflammation. This knowledge empowers you to make dietary decisions that foster a healthier, more balanced inflammatory response, setting the stage for better overall health.

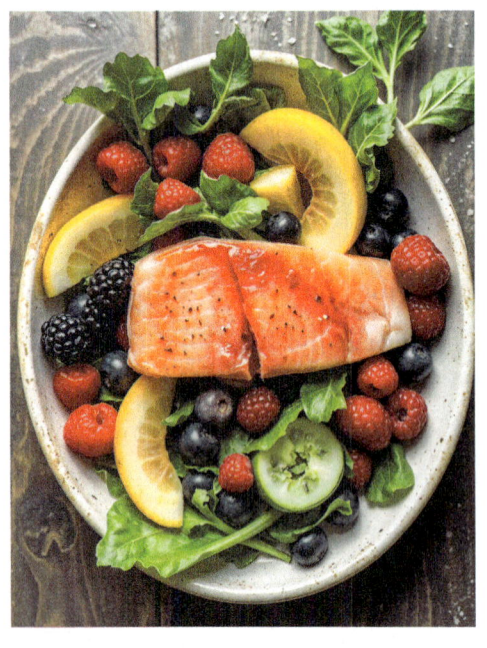

ESSENTIAL ANTI-INFLAMMATORY FOODS TO INCLUDE IN YOUR DIET

Not every food group is the same when it comes to reducing inflammation. Some have potent properties because they are abundant in vitamins, minerals, and antioxidants, which reduce inflammation and maintain optimal bodily function. Imagine your kitchen as a garden where everything you plant benefits your body in its fight against inflammation. Among the most powerful are leafy greens, berries, and fatty fish—each packed with unique properties that help dampen inflammatory processes. Leafy greens like spinach, kale, and Swiss chard are rich in vitamins A, C, E,

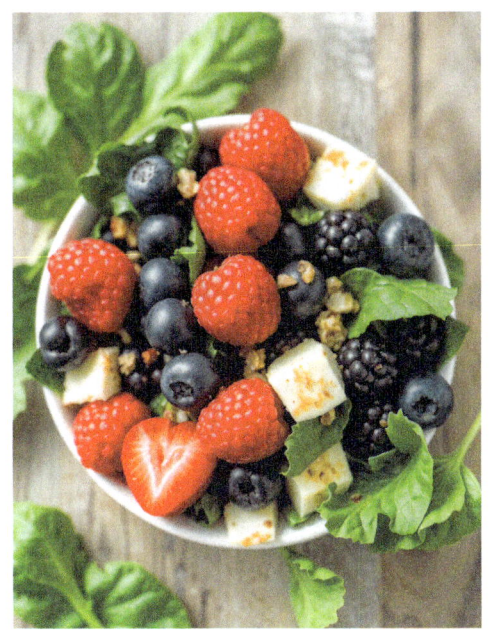

and K and minerals like iron and calcium, which are crucial for maintaining healthy cells and bodily functions. They also have a lot of antioxidants, which aid the body in fighting off damaging free radicals and lessening oxidative stress, which can cause chronic inflammation.

Meanwhile, berries aren't just delicious; they're also incredibly rich in antioxidants such as anthocyanins, giving them vibrant colors. These compounds reduce inflammation and lower the possibility of contracting long-term conditions, including diabetes and heart disease. Blueberries, strawberries, raspberries—each has its own set of flavonoids and phytochemicals contributing to their anti-inflammatory effects. Then, you'll find omega-3 fatty acid-rich fatty fish, including sardines, mackerel, and salmon. Omega-3s are fats your body can't make itself but are essential for reducing inflammation. A diet high in these fats has been linked to decreased levels of pro-inflammatory indicators such as C-reactive protein (CRP) in the blood.

Phytochemicals, too, play a starring role in managing inflammation. These compounds, which plants produce as defense mechanism, provide significant health benefits when consumed. They have anti-inflammatory properties and are associated with a decreased risk of chronic illnesses like diabetes and heart disease.

Another, kaempferol, which is prevalent in kale, gives this leafy green its anti-inflammatory, antioxidant, and anti-cancer properties. These substances are not just incidental bonuses but integral to bolstering the body's ability to fight inflammation.

Incorporating spices and herbs like ginger, turmeric, and garlic into your diet is another excellent way to combat inflammation. Turmeric, for example, contains curcumin, a compound with potent anti-inflammatory properties that matches the efficacy of some anti-inflammatory drugs but without the side effects.

It's the reason turmeric has a bright, golden color. Ginger, on the other hand, not only adds a zesty flavor to dishes but also works similarly to non-steroidal anti-inflammatory drugs by blocking inflammatory processes in the body. And then there's garlic, which has been used for years to treat various illnesses due to its anti-inflammatory and immune-boosting properties in different cultures.

Lastly, the types of fats you include in your diet can significantly impact inflammation. It's not just about reducing fat intake but choosing the right fats. Trans fats and certain saturated fats can worsen inflammation. They should be limited, but monounsaturated fats in avocados and polyunsaturated fats in nuts and seeds can help reduce them. Avocados are particularly beneficial, offering heart-healthy fats and compounds that reduce inflammation in young skin cells. Similarly, nuts like almonds and walnuts are high in omega-3 fatty acids, which help lower levels of inflammation throughout the body.

By making these foods a regular part of your diet, you're not just eating to satisfy hunger; you're actively helping your body manage inflammation. This focuses on incorporating various delicious, health-promoting foods into your meals, working synergistically to reduce inflammation rather than following a strict diet. Whether it's by blending berries into your morning smoothie, tossing some leafy greens into a salad, adding a piece of fatty fish to your dinner plate, or spicing up your meals with turmeric and ginger, each meal offers a new chance to provide your body with the nutrition it requires to combat inflammation. As your understanding of these foods and their benefits grows, you'll find it increasingly enjoyable and satisfying to make choices that taste good and are also good for your body.

FOODS TO AVOID: WHAT TRIGGERS INFLAMMATION?

Navigating the world of food can often feel like trying to find your way through a dense forest. Some foods nourish and protect your body, acting like guides and helpers, while others can potentially set off alarms, triggering inflammation. It's crucial to know which foods might be causing more harm than good, especially when aiming to reduce inflammation. Let's discuss some of the usual suspects known to provoke inflammatory responses and why limiting or avoiding them in your diet might be wise.

First, let's talk about trans fats, high-fructose corn syrup, and refined carbohydrates. These are not just buzzwords thrown around by health enthusiasts; their impact on your body is natural and often quite harmful. Trans fats are particularly notorious. They are produced by mixing vegetable oil with hydrogen, making them less likely to spoil. These fats are found in many processed foods, baked goods, and margarines. Convenient for manufacturers, yes, but not so much for your body. Consuming these fats has been linked to increased levels of harmful LDL cholesterol in the bloodstream and reduced beneficial HDL cholesterol, contributing to inflammation and heart disease.

Similarly, high-fructose corn syrup, a common sweetener in sodas, sweets, and even bread, can cause obesity, increased blood pressure, insulin resistance, and type 2 diabetes, all of which are inflammatory conditions. White bread and pastries are refined carbohydrates that can raise blood sugar levels and induce inflammation, particularly in the digestive system. Then there's the topic of dairy and red meat. While not everyone needs to avoid these (and they can be part of a healthy diet for many), people with certain health conditions may find that these foods exacerbate inflammation. Dairy products and red meats contain high levels of saturated fats, which can trigger fat tissue inflammation, a significant contributor to the development of heart disease. Preservatives known as nitrates, linked to heightened inflammation and an increased risk of chronic illness, are frequently found in processed meats like sausages and hot dogs. If you feel bloated, gassy, or uncomfortable after consuming these products, consider exploring whether you have sensitivities to them or reducing their intake to see if your symptoms improve.

Moving on to beverages, alcohol and caffeine might also affect your body's inflammatory response more than you think. Regular, excessive consumption of alcohol can weaken liver function and disrupt other multi-organ interactions, leading to systemic inflammation. However, a diet high in coffee can increase cortisol levels, leading to inflammation and stress over time. Coffee contains high levels of antioxidants and polyphenols, which make modest to moderate amounts of the beverage beneficial. Like everything in life, moderation is key.

Lastly, let's touch on food sensitivities, which are not uncommon and can significantly impact inflammation and overall health. Common sensitivities include gluten and lactose in wheat and dairy products, respectively. These sensitivities can lead to inflammatory responses in the gut, ranging from mild bloating and gas to more severe conditions, such as celiac disease or lactose intolerance. Understanding and respecting your body's limits with certain foods is crucial. It might involve some trial and error and perhaps even food sensitivity testing, but determining if you have food sensitivities can be a game-changer in managing inflammation.

By monitoring your intake of these foods and noticing how your body reacts to them, you can make more informed decisions that help lower your body's inflammatory response. It's all about creating a diet that works uniquely for you and supports rather than disrupts your health. Remember, what you eat can be your best medicine or your slowest poison. Choose wisely, listen to your body, and adjust as necessary.

READING LABELS: IDENTIFYING HIDDEN INFLAMMATORY INGREDIENTS

Occasionally, navigating the grocery store's aisles might resemble working as a detective on a case, particularly when attempting to stay clear of the inflammatory substances frequently disguised in packaged goods. It's not just about preventing obvious culprits like sugar or fat; it's about understanding the subtle ways these and other ingredients can be listed on labels, making them less noticeable to the untrained eye. Let's break down the essentials of reading food labels so you can make informed choices that align with your anti-inflammatory goals. This knowledge turns a routine shopping trip into a powerful act of self-care.

Firstly, decoding food labels is essential beyond just glancing at the calorie count. Manufacturers often use various names for sugars and unhealthy fats to make their products appear healthier. For example, sugar can appear as high-fructose corn syrup, cane sugar, inverted sugar, or even something as benign-sounding as fruit juice concentrate. These are all sugars, and excess consumption can contribute to inflammation. Similarly, manufacturers might list trans fats as partially hydrogenated oils, which won't raise a red flag unless you know what to look for. Becoming familiar with these terms is like learning a new language—the language of labels—which empowers you to make choices that better support your health.

Moreover, it's crucial to spot and understand the role of additives and preservatives, which can be significant players in the inflammation game. Common culprits include monosodium glutamate (MSG), artificial sweeteners like aspartame, and various food colorings. Manufacturers often include these additives to enhance flavor, preserve texture, or improve color. However, for some people, they can trigger inflammatory responses, such as headaches, digestive upset, or worse, depending on individual sensitivities. Recognizing these ingredients on labels can help you avoid unnecessary discomfort and keep your anti-inflammatory diet on track.

Now, let's talk about practical shopping tips. A good rule of thumb in the supermarket is to favor whole and unprocessed foods—think fresh fruits and vegetables, bulk nuts and seeds, and fresh meats and fish—over canned or prepared items. These foods are the foundation of an anti-inflammatory diet and are less likely to contain the hidden ingredients that can sabotage your health efforts. However, opt for those with the shortest ingredient lists when packaged products are necessary. A long list often indicates the presence of unnecessary additives and preservatives. Additionally, try to shop the store's perimeter as much as possible. The freshest foods are typically displayed here, while the inner aisles contain more processed items.

Adopting these practices might seem daunting initially, but it becomes second nature with some persistence and practice. Remember, every label you read and understand is a step toward better health and well-being. By educating yourself about the ingredients in your food, you're taking control of your diet and, by extension, your inflammatory responses. This proactive approach helps reduce inflammation and contributes to a greater understanding of how food affects your body, leading to more mindful and healthy eating habits.

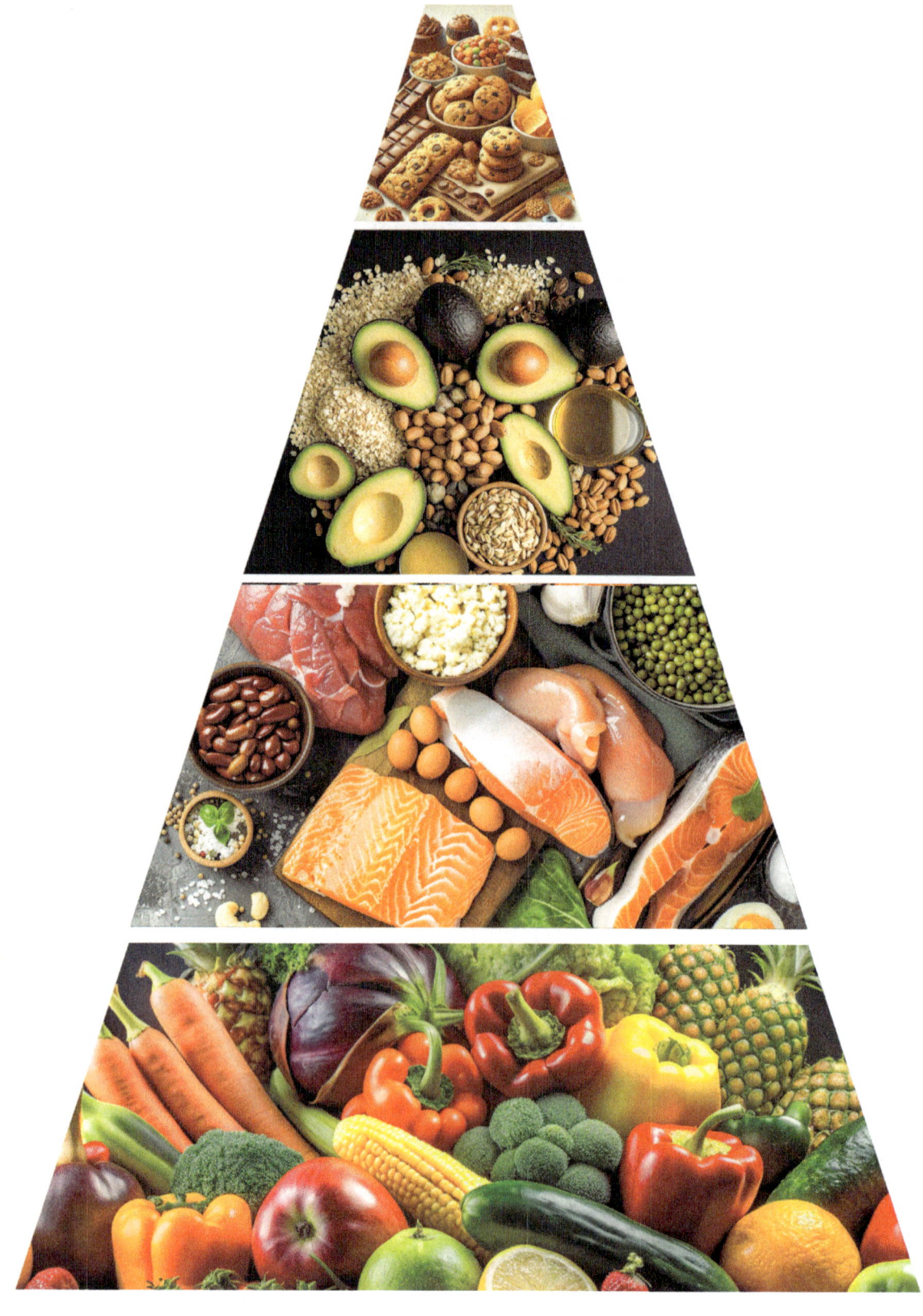

THE ANTI-INFLAMMATORY FOOD PYRAMID EXPLAINED

Imagine your diet as a building, where each brick represents a type of food. Your diet should promote a healthy, anti-inflammatory lifestyle, just as a strong building needs a solid foundation. The Anti-Inflammatory Food Pyramid is a straightforward visual guide for structuring your diet to help control inflammation and promote overall health. The pyramid is tailored specifically for those looking to reduce inflammation. Each level represents different types of foods and their recommended intake.

You'll find vegetables and fruits at the pyramid's base—the most significant and fundamental layer. It's not just about tossing a few lettuce leaves on your plate; it's about making these nutrient-rich powerhouses the foundation of your diet. Think of filling at least half your plate with various vegetables and fruits at each meal. Why is there such a focus here? Vegetables and fruits naturally lower inflammation since they are rich in vitamins, minerals, and antioxidants. They're also incredibly versatile. Their distinct anti-inflammatory qualities and intriguing aromas enhance leafy greens like spinach and kale and vibrant berries and citrus fruits. Daily, aim for four to five servings each, where a serving might look like a cup of leafy vegetables or a medium-sized piece of fruit.

The next level up the pyramid highlights proteins. Protein is crucial for repairing tissues and maintaining muscle mass, but the type of protein you choose can affect your inflammatory levels. Plant-based proteins like beans, lentils, and tofu are excellent choices as they're low in fat, high in fiber, and other nutrients, helping curb inflammation. Lean animal proteins, mainly fish like salmon and mackerel, are also beneficial due to their high omega-3 fatty acid content, which makes them potent anti-inflammatory agents. Poultry like chicken and turkey provide suitable alternatives, but skinless versions are preferred to minimize saturated fat intake. Integrating various protein sources throughout your week supports your dietary goals and keeps your meals interesting.

As we approach the top of the pyramid, we find fats—a more minor but essential part of the diet. However, not all fats are created equal. Focus on incorporating healthy fats that support anti-inflammatory processes. These include the monounsaturated fats in avocados, nuts, and olive oil and the polyunsaturated fats in seeds and fatty fish. These fats are good for reducing inflammation and helping absorb vitamins in other foods consumed during the meal, enhancing overall nutritional intake. However, moderation is vital, as all fats are calorie-dense.

At the very top of the pyramid—the most minor portion—reside those foods that someone should consume sparingly. This category includes processed foods and items high in refined sugars and saturated fats.

It's about something other than eliminating these from your diet, which can be unrealistic and unsustainable. Instead, know these are not everyday foods and should be treated as occasional indulgences. Processed snacks, sweets, and fast food often contain trans fats and sugars that can trigger inflammatory responses, so limiting these helps control inflammation and promote better health.

Understanding this pyramid structure is like having a map that guides you toward making choices that fit within a healthy, anti-inflammatory eating pattern. It's about balance and variety, ensuring each meal brings something beneficial to your table and supports your body's fight against inflammation. As you grow accustomed to this eating method, you'll find it second nature. You'll start to notice how different foods affect your body, adjusting your diet to maximize your health and well-being without feeling restricted. This approach helps manage inflammation and enriches your diet with a spectrum of flavors and nutrients, making each meal a step toward a healthier life.

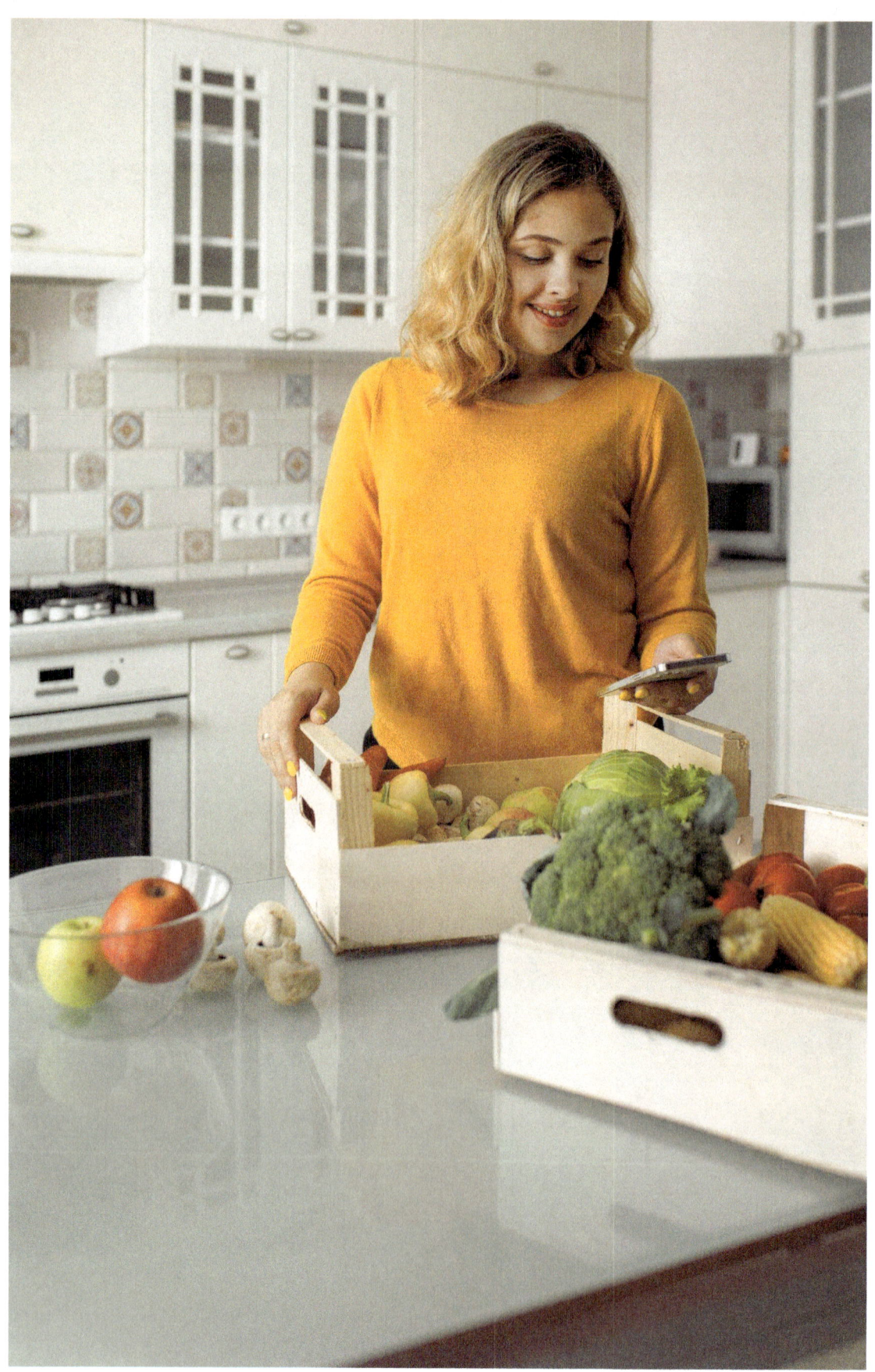

2

SETTING UP FOR SUCCESS ON YOUR DIET JOURNEY

Imagine walking into your kitchen and feeling a sense of calm and control, knowing that everything in this space will help you succeed on your anti-inflammatory diet. It sounds great. Well, it's achievable! A kitchen makeover isn't just about aesthetics; it's about transforming your environment to support your health goals. Let's explore how you can organize and equip your kitchen to make sticking to an anti-inflammatory diet more accessible and enjoyable.

KITCHEN MAKEOVER: PREPARING YOUR SPACE FOR SUCCESS

Organizing For Accessibility

The first step in your kitchen makeover is organizing for accessibility. This means setting up your kitchen so that the healthiest choices are the easiest. Start with your refrigerator. Place fruits, vegetables, and other anti-inflammatory foods at eye level. Why? Well, we often reach for what's directly in front of us. If the first thing you see when you open the fridge is a colorful array of fruits and veggies, you're more likely to choose those instead of digging around for less healthy options that might be hidden in the drawers.

Similarly, organize your cabinets and pantry so that whole grains, spices, nuts, and seeds are front and center. Consider using clear storage containers for these items to keep them fresh and make it visually simple to see what you have on hand. This visibility makes meal prep quicker (because you know exactly where everything is) and encourages you to use these nutritious ingredients more often.

Essential Kitchen Tools

Next, let's talk about the tools of the trade. Meal preparation may be easier and more fun with the appropriate tools. A high-quality blender is a must for whipping up anti-inflammatory smoothies or soups. A high-quality set of knives will make chopping those fruits and veggies a breeze, which is a game-changer if you're incorporating more plant-based foods into your diet. And don't underestimate the power of reasonable storage solutions—airtight containers are essential for keeping prepped meals fresh and preventing flavors from mingling in the fridge.

Investing in these tools doesn't have to break the bank. Consider which items you'll use most often and start there. Over time, you can build up your kitchen gadgets and utensils as you find what works best for your new eating habits.

Removing Temptations

Removing temptation is one of the most effective ways to stick to any diet. Go through your kitchen and purge it of foods heavy in trans fats, processed sugar, and artificial ingredients—all of which can contribute to inflammation. If you have family members who aren't on the same dietary page, designate a specific cabinet or shelf for their snacks so you're not constantly tempted when preparing a meal.

Initially, this may feel wasteful, but it's about setting yourself up for success. You're much less likely to snack on unhealthy options if they aren't there. Plus, it clears the way for you to stock up on healthier alternatives that support your anti-inflammatory journey.

Setting Up a Healthy Pantry

Finally, setting up a healthy pantry is like laying the foundation for your new dietary habits. Stock it with anti-inflammatory staples like whole grains (think quinoa, brown rice, and whole grain pasta), an array of spices (turmeric, ginger, and garlic are great choices), nuts, and seeds. These ingredients can be used in many recipes and have long shelf lives, making them cost-effective and convenient.

Think of your pantry as your toolbox. Each item in it should help you build delicious, nutritious meals that fight inflammation and support your overall health. Arrange these staples so they're easy to see and reach; this will encourage you to use them.

Transforming your kitchen into a space that supports your anti-inflammatory diet isn't just about physical changes; it's about setting a positive, health-focused intention. Every time you step into your kitchen, you'll feel a sense of readiness and excitement to continue on this path. The proper setup makes it easier to stick to your dietary goals and makes the process enjoyable. After all, nurturing your body should feel good, and creating a kitchen that supports it is a big step in the right direction.

BUDGET-FRIENDLY SHOPPING FOR ANTI-INFLAMMATORY INGREDIENTS

When it comes to stocking your kitchen with anti-inflammatory foods, it's natural to be concerned about the potential strain it may place on your budget. After all, fresh, high-quality ingredients often come with a higher price tag, right? Well, not necessarily. There are plenty of strategies to keep your shopping budget-friendly while still packing your pantry with nutritious options that help fend off inflammation. Let's walk through some savvy shopping tips that won't break the bank but will definitely enrich your diet.

One of the most effective ways to shop smart is by buying fruits and vegetables that are in season. Not only does this practice reduce costs, but it also ensures that you're getting produce packed with optimal flavor and nutrients. Seasonal produce has yet to travel long distances, which often compromises both taste and nutritional value. For instance, buying strawberries in the summer and squash in the fall can lead to savings at the checkout and add a delicious, healthy variety to your meals. If you need clarification on what's in season, a brief web search or a conversation with nearby farmers at the market can guide you. This practice can turn your meal planning into a seasonal adventure that's both fun and good for your body.

Now, let's discuss bulk buying, which can be especially advantageous for staples like whole grains, nuts, and seeds—key components of an anti-inflammatory diet. Many stores offer bulk bins, which not only help reduce packaging waste but also allow you to buy precisely the amount you need, potentially lowering your overall costs. Buying in bulk typically ensures a lower price per unit; you can store these staples for a long time without spoilage. Think of items like quinoa, almonds, and flaxseeds—versatile ingredients that can be used in many recipes. Properly storing them is essential. Store them in sealed containers in a cold, dark place to preserve their freshness and nutrient value. Exploring local markets and joining a Community-Supported Agriculture (CSA) program are other fantastic ways to support your anti-inflammatory diet economically. Local farmers' markets often offer organic produce at lower prices than you might find at grocery stores, and because the produce is local, it's fresh and packed with maximum nutrients. CSA programs take this further by allowing you to buy a share of a local farm's produce for the season. Every box of fresh fruits and vegetables contains produce picked at its peak ripeness. Every week or two supports local farmers and pushes you to get creative with whatever is seasonal and fresh.

Lastly, pay attention to the power of choosing generic brands for certain staples like spices, oils, and canned goods. These products often match their brand-name counterparts in quality but are more wallet-friendly. Most stores offer branded savings programs to help you save money on grocery bills without sacrificing quality. For example, generic brands of olive oil or canned tomatoes can be just as good as the pump brands if you know what to look for (such as "extra virgin" on olive oil labels or "no added salt" on canned veggies).

By using these techniques when shopping, you can experience a diet rich in anti-inflammatory foods without stressing over the cost. It's all about being a savvy shopper—knowing when to buy in season, when to buy in bulk, where to find the best local produce, and when it's okay to go generic. With these tips, you can nourish your body with the best foods for fighting inflammation and keep your budget happy at the same time.

THE ART OF MEAL PREPPING: SIMPLE STEPS TO SAVE TIME

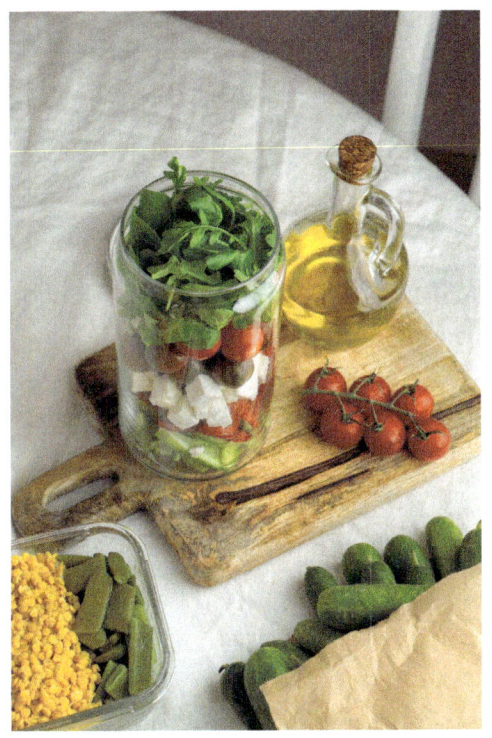

Meal prepping is like setting yourself up with little gifts throughout the week—open your fridge and find healthy, homemade meals waiting to be enjoyed. This isn't just about saving time; it's about creating a sustainable habit that supports your anti-inflammatory diet without the daily hassle. Let's walk through how to make meal prep a fun and practical part of your routine.

Planning your meals for the week might seem daunting at first, but it's a liberating process once you get the hang of it. Start by choosing a day when you have a few hours to spare— maybe a Sunday afternoon or a Wednesday evening, depending on your schedule. This will be your meal planning and preparation time. Grab a notepad or favorite meal-planning app and jot down what you'd like to eat for the week. Remember to include all meals and snacks. Variety is key to keeping things interesting, so try to mix up your dishes with different proteins, whole grains, and plenty of fresh veggies. Plan around foods you have in bulk or seasonal produce you've picked up from the market to keep things budget-friendly and fresh.

Once your menu is set, create a shopping list based on your chosen recipes. This list ensures you buy just what you need, reducing waste and unnecessary purchases. When shopping, stick to your list, but allow some flexibility for great deals on items like blueberries or a special on your favorite fish. Use these opportunities to tweak your meal plan slightly and enjoy the spontaneity that can make cooking fun.

Now, let's talk about batch cooking, a game-changer for prepping. The idea here is to cook large portions of versatile ingredients or full meals that can be eaten throughout the week. Think big pots of quinoa or rice, trays of roasted vegetables, grilled chicken breasts, or a large batch of a hearty veggie and bean chili. These are all interchangeable to produce different meals, adding variety to your diet without extra daily cooking. For instance, roasted chicken can be sliced atop a fresh salad one day, mixed into a spicy chicken wrap the next, and stirred into a comforting soup later in the week.

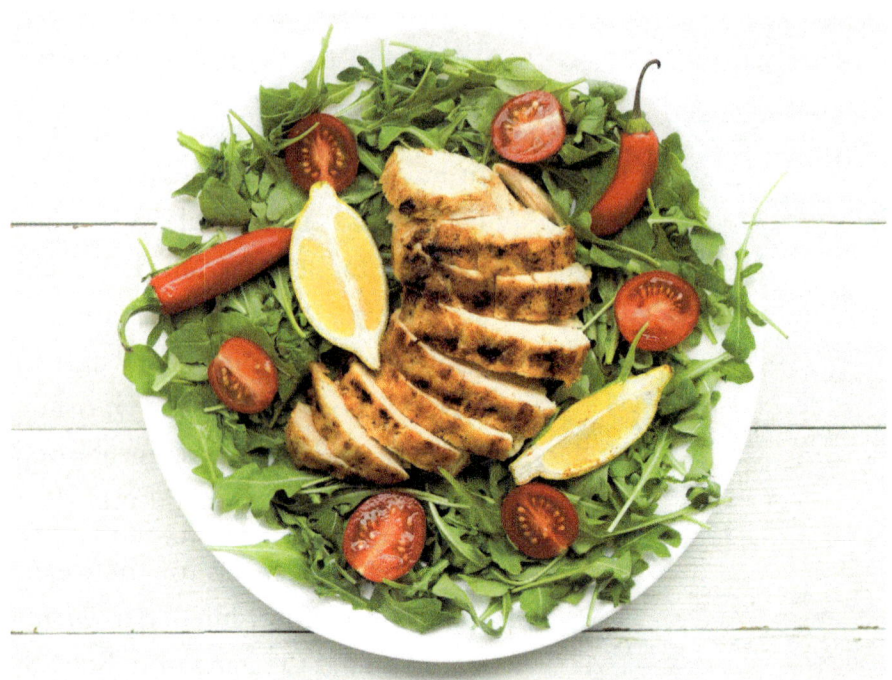

Practical batch cooking relies on some cooking techniques and appliances that save time and preserve the nutritional content of your food. Either a pressure cooker or a slow cooker can be handy here. These tools allow you to toss in many ingredients, set the timer, and walk away while they do all the work. Imagine coming home to a slow-cooked stew simmering gently, blending flavors, and tenderizing meat without supervision. Or use a pressure cooker to make a batch of beans or stew in a fraction of the time it usually takes. These methods save time and help retain the nutrients often lost during high-temperature or prolonged cooking.

Storing your prepped meals is the final step in your meal-prepping journey. Store items correctly to preserve freshness and avoid spoiling. Invest in good-quality, airtight containers, from the fridge to the microwave or oven. Glass containers are great as they don't harbor smells and are generally easier to clean than plastic. Portion your meals into individual containers, assigning one container for each meal. It's effortless to grab a container, heat it up, and enjoy a healthy meal, even on your busiest days. Keep your fridge organized so you can easily see and access your prepped meals, making reaching for something less healthy less likely.

Embracing meal prep as part of your routine might take some practice, but once you've got a system in place, you'll wonder how you ever managed without it. Not only does it help you stick to your anti-inflammatory diet by having healthy options readily available, but it also frees up your time during the week for more of what you love—all while ensuring you're nourished and well-fed. Now, isn't that a win-win?

ANTI-INFLAMMATORY COOKING TECHNIQUES TO MAXIMIZE BENEFITS

When discussing an anti-inflammatory diet, we often focus on what to eat. Equally important, however, is how you prepare your food. Your chosen method significantly impacts the nutritional punch your meals pack and their ability to help combat inflammation. Let's explore some cooking techniques to help you get the most out of your anti-inflammatory ingredients, ensuring that every bite you take supports your health.

Steaming and poaching are two of the gentlest ways to cook food, helping to preserve the precious nutrients that can be lost through other, more intense cooking methods. Steaming involves cooking food in a basket suspended above simmering water; it's a fantastic way to prepare vegetables as it helps maintain their color, texture, and, most importantly, their vitamins and minerals. Broccoli, for example, keeps its glorious green hue and crispness, along with its cancer-fighting compounds like sulforaphane, which can be diminished by overcooking. Poaching, which involves gently simmering food in a small amount of water or broth, is ideal for delicate items like fish or eggs. This method not only preserves the flavor and texture but also ensures that the omega-3 fatty acids in fish, crucial for fighting inflammation, are not damaged by high heat.

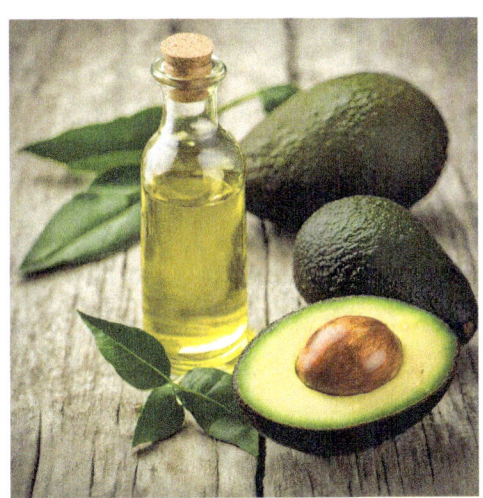

The oils you choose and how you use them are pivotal in an anti-inflammatory kitchen. Olive oil and avocado oil are among your best bets. Rich in monounsaturated fats, these oils assist in lowering unhealthy cholesterol levels and decreasing cardiovascular risk when used in moderation. However, it's crucial to avoid smoking the oil, which happens when it's heated beyond its smoke point and begins to break down, potentially forming harmful compounds and losing some beneficial properties. For instance, olive oil smokes at a lower temperature than avocado oil, making it better suited for light sautéing or adding to dishes after cooking. On the other hand, avocado oil, with its higher smoke point, is great for cooking at slightly higher temperatures. Remember, the key is to use these oils wisely to leverage their anti-inflammatory benefits without compromising their integrity.

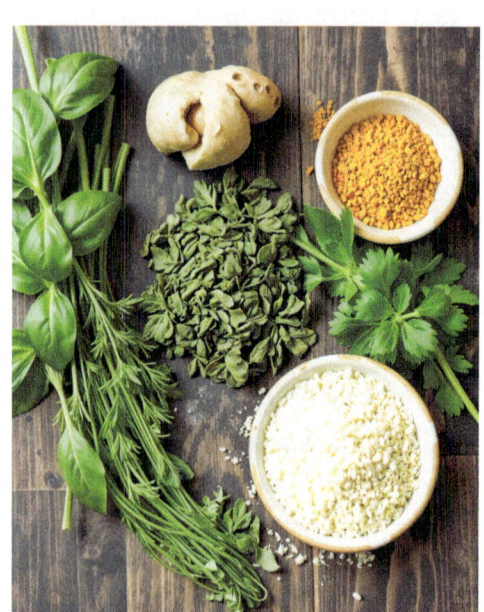

Herbs and spices are flavor enhancers and rich in anti-inflammatory properties. Curcumin, the key ingredient in turmeric, has been proven to reduce metabolic syndrome and arthritis-related inflammation. Start integrating turmeric into your cooking, beginning with a pinch in smoothies or rice dishes and gradually increasing as you become accustomed to the flavor. Similarly, ginger, used in everything from teas to stir-fry dishes, can help alleviate muscle pain and soreness with its anti-inflammatory effects. Remember about garlic? Beyond its ability to elevate any dish, garlic has been celebrated for its immune-boosting and anti-inflammatory properties. Making these spices staples in your kitchen allows you to season your dishes generously, boosting your taste and health.

Lastly, the temperature at which you cook can make a big difference. High-heat methods like frying or grilling can create advanced glycation end products (AGEs) and other harmful compounds that can trigger inflammation. Instead, opt for lower temperatures and slower cooking methods as often as possible. Slow cooking, for instance, deepens flavors and cooks meats and vegetables at low temperatures, reducing the formation of harmful compounds and preserving nutrients. This method also allows for the better breakdown of tough fibers in meat and vegetables, making them easier to digest and their nutrients more accessible.

By adopting these cooking methods, you can make your meals more delicious and transform your kitchen into a hub for health promotion. These techniques ensure that the integrity of your ingredients is maintained, maximizing their anti-inflammatory potential and allowing you to enjoy every meal confident that you are nourishing your body in the best ways possible.

MANAGING DINING OUT—MAKING SMART CHOICES

Eating out doesn't have to be a daunting task when you're following an anti-inflammatory diet. With some know-how and preparation, you can enjoy restaurant meals without straying from your health goals. Let's start with selecting the right places to eat. Becoming a restaurant detective before you leave the house is a great idea. Many restaurants now offer their menus online, allowing you to scope the options in advance. Look for places that emphasize fresh, whole foods and have a variety of vegetable-heavy dishes. Restaurants catering to specific dietary needs or highlighting their use of local and organic produce is often a good bet. If the menu is not available online, please call ahead and ask about their offerings. Most chefs are more than willing to accommodate guests trying to eat healthily.

Once you've chosen a restaurant, the next step is tailoring your order to meet your specific dietary requirements. It's much easier than it sounds. Start by scanning the menu for dishes that are close to what you need. Salads, grilled entrees, and vegetable sides can usually be adapted easily. Feel free to request dressings or sauces on the side and ask for any fried menu items to be grilled. Double-check the ingredients if you choose a salad; even a salad can hide inflammatory items like fried or creamy dressings. Substituting these with olive oil, lemon juice, or vinegar can be a simple yet effective way to control inflammation.

The regulation of portion size is still another essential factor when dining out. Restaurant portions are often much more significant than we need, and eating more than intended is easy when a full plate is in front of us. You can tackle this in a few ways. Consider offering a dinner companion a meal to share or asking the server to box up half of the entree before it comes to the table. Not only does this help you manage your portion size, but it also means you have a delicious leftover meal for the next day! Smaller plates or appetizer portions can also be a good choice, particularly if you want to try a bit of everything without overdoing it.

Let's talk about beverages, as they can also be a hidden source of sugar and other inflammatory agents. Sugary sodas, certain alcoholic drinks, and even some fruit juices can undermine your efforts to stick to an anti-inflammatory diet. Opting for water is always a safe bet, and it helps to stay hydrated. If you want something more exciting, ask for a spritz of lemon or lime in your water. Herbal teas are another excellent choice, and many have anti-inflammatory properties. If you drink alcohol, opt for a glass of red wine or a clear liquor mixed with a splash of a simple mixer-like tonic water. Avoid cocktails heavy on sugar or premade mixes, as they often contain hidden inflammatory ingredients.

Navigating dining out while keeping your anti-inflammatory goals in check is about making informed choices. With these tips, you can enjoy social outings and delicious meals without compromising your health. Remember, it's about balance and making the best options available. Whether choosing the right restaurant, customizing your order, managing portion sizes, or selecting healthier beverages, you have the tools to maintain your anti-inflammatory diet wherever you go.

ADDRESSING COMMON DIET TRANSITION CHALLENGES

Switching to an anti-inflammatory diet can feel easy on some days and challenging on others, especially when cravings hit or you're navigating social settings. Adjusting your eating habits is a significant change, and it's perfectly normal to encounter a few bumps along the way. Here are some strategies to help you manage these challenges effectively, keeping you on track toward your health goals.

Cravings for sugary or fatty foods can be one of the most challenging hurdles. It's important to acknowledge these cravings rather than ignore them. Often, they signal that your body is adjusting to new dietary habits. One effective strategy is finding healthy alternatives. If you're craving something sweet, try reaching for a banana, another type of fruit, or a small serving of dark chocolate instead of the usual cookie or candy bar. If it's the crunch of chips you miss, try a handful of nuts or some air-popped popcorn. Sometimes, cravings can also be a sign of dehydration, so drinking a glass of water might be surprisingly effective. Remember, it's okay to indulge occasionally. Allowing yourself a treat can help keep you from feeling deprived and may prevent overindulgence later.

Social gatherings and family meals can also pose challenges, particularly when the menu aligns differently with your dietary choices. A good approach is to bring a dish to share that fits within your eating plan. Not only does this ensure you have something to enjoy, but it also introduces your friends and family to the delicious possibilities of anti-inflammatory eating. Please communicate your dietary needs to your host; most will accommodate. Additionally, focus on the social aspect of these gatherings. Enjoy the company and conversation, which can make the specifics of food less central to the experience.

Maintaining motivation can wane, especially after the initial excitement wears off. To keep your spirits high, consider keeping a food journal. Tracking what you eat, how you feel, and the improvements you're noticing can reinforce the benefits of your dietary changes. Setting small, achievable goals can also provide a sense of accomplishment. Maybe this week, you aim to try two new anti-inflammatory recipes or master a handmade take on your preferred takeout meal.

Additionally, joining a support group, whether online or in person, can connect you with others on similar paths. Hearing other people's stories and advice can be immensely uplifting and reassuring. Educating others about your dietary choices can sometimes feel tricky, especially if you encounter skepticism or curiosity from friends and family. Approach these conversations with openness and positivity. Share your reasons for choosing this diet, focusing on the personal benefits you've experienced or hope to achieve. Offering to cook a meal or sharing articles and books explaining the science behind anti-inflammatory eating can help others understand your choices. Remember, this isn't about convincing anyone to join you but seeking their support and respect for your decisions.

These strategies aren't just about overcoming challenges and embracing and enjoying your new dietary habits. Each hurdle you clear reinforces your commitment and builds your confidence, proving that you can make lasting changes for your health. As you continue to navigate these challenges, remember that each day brings new opportunities to nourish your body and well-being.

As we wrap up this chapter on setting up for success in your anti-inflammatory diet journey, remember that the change encompasses more than just changing what's on your plate. It's about adapting your lifestyle to embrace new eating habits, handling cravings, social situations, and motivational dips, and effectively communicating your needs to those around you. These foundational steps pave the way for a smoother transition, ensuring you can stick to your goals and thrive on this new path. With your kitchen now optimized for healthy cooking, your savvy shopping skills and meal-prepping techniques in place, and a solid strategy for facing common challenges, you're well-equipped to continue this adventure.

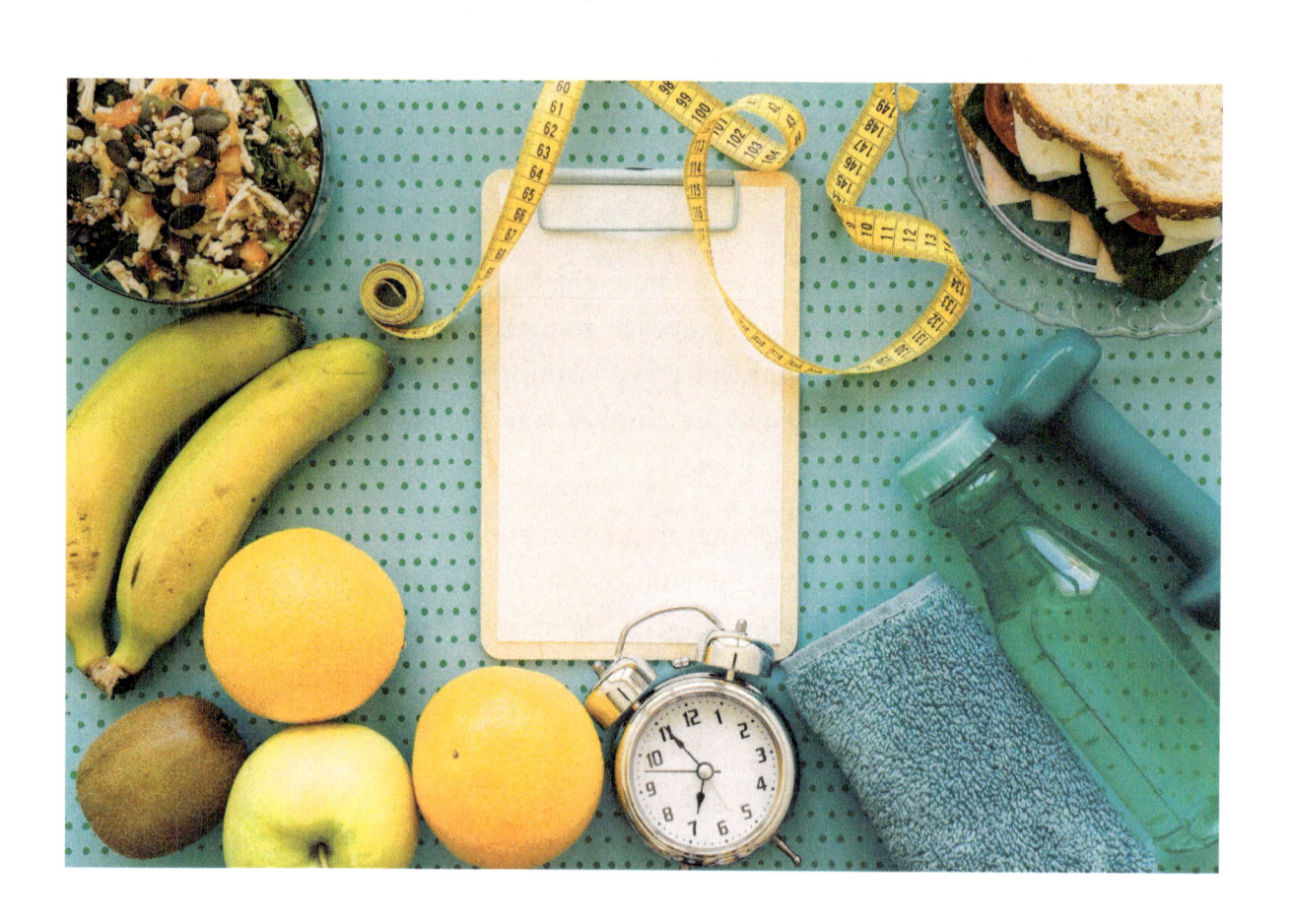

3

WEIGHT MANAGEMENT AND NUTRITIONAL INSIGHTS

Imagine stepping onto a scale and feeling a sense of achievement—not because of the number, but because you feel healthier, more energetic, and lighter. It's a familiar scene many dream about but often struggle to achieve. Yet, what if I told you that managing your weight could be more about the quality of the foods you eat than the quantity? This chapter explores how an anti-inflammatory diet can help you manage weight and enhance general health.

THE ROLE OF AN ANTI-INFLAMMATORY DIET IN WEIGHT LOSS

Have you ever considered that your body's inflammatory response might affect your weight? It's a connection that often goes unnoticed. Chronic inflammation can significantly influence your body's metabolism and fat storage. For instance, increased inflammation can affect insulin, the hormone responsible for regulating blood sugar levels. When your body starts to resist insulin due to chronic inflammation, it can lead to higher blood sugar levels, making weight loss more challenging. Similarly, inflammation can affect another hormone, leptin, which is crucial for regulating hunger and energy expenditure. Inflammation can disrupt leptin signals, making you feel hungry even when your body doesn't need more food.

Now, let's talk about the food itself. Anti-inflammatory diets are rich in nutrients and low in processed foods, focusing heavily on vegetables, fruits, whole grains, and lean proteins. These foods are naturally lower in calories yet rich in fiber, which helps you feel full longer. For example, a meal could be as simple as a grilled chicken breast, a side of quinoa, and a heaping serving of steamed broccoli—a filling that is nutrient-rich and lower in calories than many processed options. The broccoli fiber helps fill you up and stabilizes your blood sugar, preventing the spikes and crashes that can lead to overeating.

Moreover, adopting an anti-inflammatory diet doesn't mean you have to feel deprived. It's about making smarter food choices that contribute to weight loss and enhancing overall health. For example, swapping out a bowl of sugary cereal for oatmeal topped with fresh berries and a sprinkle of cinnamon can significantly reduce inflammation and control calorie intake. These changes are sustainable and beneficial, helping to shift your eating habits gradually and effectively.

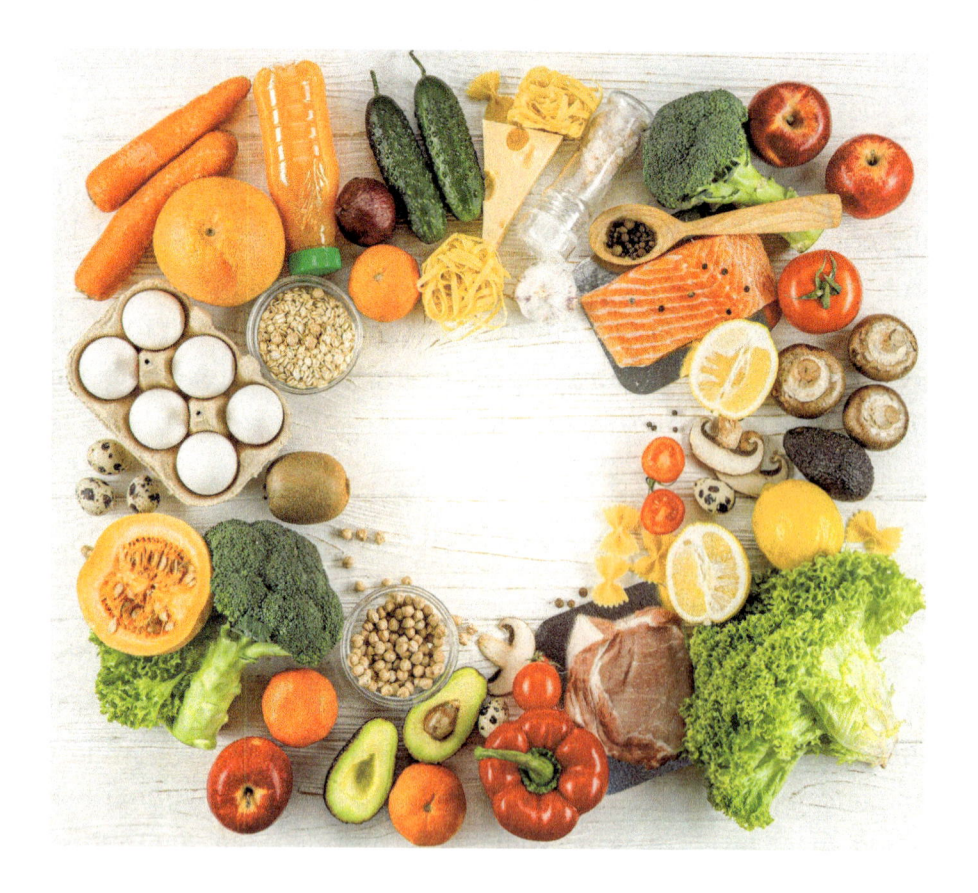

To bring this to life, consider the story of Sarah (name changed for privacy), a thirty-five-year-old who struggled with her weight for years. After shifting to an anti-inflammatory diet, not only did she lose significant weight, but she also experienced increased energy and reduced joint pain. Her success came not from counting every calorie but from focusing on rich, nutritious foods that naturally supported her body's needs. Sarah's story is just one of many that highlight the practical benefits and transformative potential of integrating an anti-inflammatory approach into one's lifestyle.

Embracing an anti-inflammatory diet for weight management is more than just shedding pounds; it's about fostering a healthier relationship with food. It encourages you to look beyond the calorie content and focus on the nutritional value, leading to better choices that support your body's natural processes. This approach helps reduce weight and enhances overall well-being, making it a rewarding path for anyone looking to improve their health.

UNDERSTANDING CALORIES AND MACRONUTRIENTS IN YOUR DIET

Let's unravel the mystery of calories and macronutrients, which are pivotal in effectively managing an anti-inflammatory diet. Think of calories as little packets of energy; your body needs them to perform everything from breathing to jogging. Each activity consumes energy, and the calories you eat fuel these activities. However, not all calories are created equal. Depending on where they come from—carbohydrates, proteins, or fats—each serves a unique function in your body.

Carbohydrates, proteins, and fats, collectively known as macronutrients, play unique roles in your diet. Carbohydrates are your body's primary energy source. The body converts carbohydrates into glucose, a sugar that powers your tissues, organs, and cells. They are essential if you lead an active lifestyle because they provide quick energy. Proteins, on the other hand, are the building blocks of your body. They help repair tissues, make enzymes and hormones, and are essential in maintaining muscle mass and a healthy immune system. Then there are fats, often misunderstood but crucial. Healthy fats help absorb vitamins, provide energy, support cell growth, and protect your organs. They also play a vital role in managing inflammation; omega-3 fatty acids, found in foods like fish and flaxseeds, are particularly good at this.

Calculating your daily caloric needs can sound like a math puzzle, but it's straightforward with the right tools. Various factors, such as age, gender, activity level, and personal health goals (like losing, maintaining, or gaining weight), play into this equation. Numerous calculators are available online where you input your details, and they tell you how many calories you should consume daily. This personalized number helps guide your food choices and portion sizes, fueling your body optimally without overeating or undereating.

The balance of these macronutrients can also influence inflammation in your body. For instance, diets high in refined carbs and bad fats can spur inflammation, while those rich in omega-3 fatty acids and fiber can help reduce it. Let's say you're adjusting your diet to manage inflammation. You might consider lowering your intake of saturated fats and increasing your omega-3s. It applies not only to the types of foods you eat but also to their ratios.

Perhaps your diet involves more healthy fats and proteins while keeping your carb intake lower and focused on complex carbs, which have a slower release of energy and don't spike your blood sugar levels.

Understanding these nutritional fundamentals allows for better inflammation management and a more balanced and healthy approach to eating. Knowing how your body processes different foods and adjusting your diet to accommodate your energy needs can significantly impact how you feel and function daily. This approach is not just about cutting out certain food types; it's about creating a balanced plate that supports your body's unique needs, helping you feel your best both inside and out.

BALANCING CARBS, PROTEINS, AND FATS

When you're refining your diet to quell inflammation and manage weight, understanding the balancing act between carbohydrates, proteins, and fats can be a game-changer. It's like being a DJ at a party; you need to mix the right tracks to keep the vibe upbeat and pleasant. Let's break down how you can create harmony with these macronutrients to keep your body humming healthily.

The focus on carbohydrates should be on selecting complex carbs over simple carbs, starting with carbohydrates. It's not just about choosing brown rice over white rice; it's about understanding why.

Complex carbohydrates, such as whole grains, legumes, and a broad array of vegetables, break down slowly in your body. This slow digestion process helps maintain steady blood sugar levels, avoiding the spikes that simple carbohydrates often induce. These spikes are not just harmful to your mood and energy levels; they can exacerbate inflammatory responses in your body. Foods rich in complex carbohydrates are also high in fiber, which helps reduce inflammation by promoting digestive health and regulating immune functions. So, next time you're meal planning, consider incorporating a serving of quinoa or a hearty bean stew. These aren't just filling; they're working in the background to keep inflammation in check.

Proteins, your body's building blocks, are crucial not just for muscle repair and growth but also for supporting overall health, including managing inflammation. The trick is to choose your protein sources wisely. Anti-inflammatory proteins provide the building blocks without the inflammatory side effects that some high-fat meats might elicit. Great choices include fatty fish like salmon and mackerel, which are rich in omega-3 fatty acids known for their anti-inflammatory properties. Plant-based proteins such as lentils, chickpeas, and tofu offer ample protein and provide additional nutrients like fiber and minerals, enhancing their health benefits. Including a variety of these proteins in your diet will provide all the amino acids and other nutrients your body needs for metabolic and repair activities. Now, let's talk about fat. The world of dietary fats is vast, but here's the gist: saturated and trans fats are wrong, and unsaturated fats are good. Saturated fats, found in things like butter and certain cuts of meat, can trigger fat tissue inflammation, which is not what you want when trying to keep inflammation at bay. Trans fats are considerably worse and are frequently included in processed foods, as they can increase harmful cholesterol levels and lower good cholesterol, leading to inflammation. Instead, focus on unsaturated fats, particularly those in olive oil, nuts, and avocados. These fats are not only heart-healthy but also beneficial for reducing inflammation. They help absorb essential vitamins and protect your cells from damage—think of them as your body's peacekeepers, keeping inflammation under control.

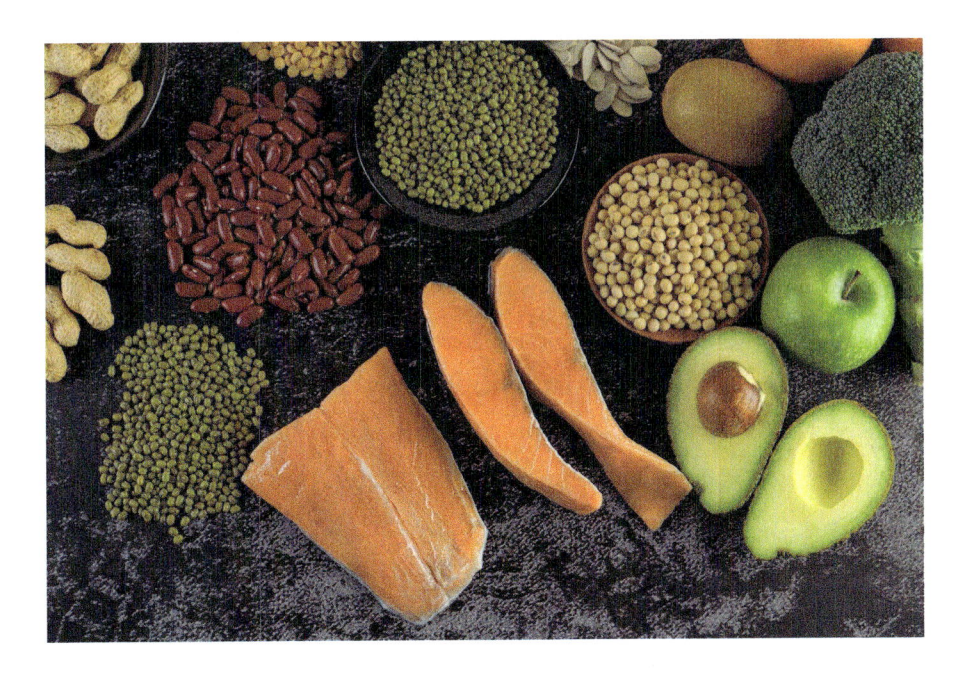

Putting all these pieces together in a meal might seem complex, but it's pretty simple once you get the hang of it. The key is balance. Lean protein, healthy fats, and a solid quantity of complex carbs are the components of a well-rounded meal. For instance, a dinner plate could feature grilled salmon (protein and healthy fat), a side of quinoa (complex carb), and a vibrant salad tossed with olive oil (more healthy fat). This combination satisfies your taste buds and provides a balanced mix of nutrients that work together to reduce inflammation and promote overall health.

Embracing this balanced approach to macronutrients isn't just about reducing inflammation or managing weight; it's about setting the stage for long-term health. By choosing your carbs, proteins, and fats wisely, you're not just eating; you're curating a diet that continuously contributes to your well-being. Always remember that managing your meal balance is crucial to supporting your body's natural functions and providing nourishment at every meal. As you become more familiar with these principles, you'll find it easier to make choices that naturally align with your body's needs, leading to improved health and vitality.

NUTRIENT-DENSE FOODS TO ENHANCE MEAL QUALITY

When we talk about nutrient-dense foods, we're referring to foods that pack a lot of vitamins, minerals, antioxidants, and other health-promoting substances into each calorie. These are the superheroes of your diet, providing your body with essential nutrients without many empty calories. Think of kale, berries, and salmon as prime examples. Kale is a leafy green powerhouse packed with vitamins A, C, and K and minerals like manganese and calcium, all with minimal calories. Berries, such as blueberries and strawberries, are not just delicious; they're also rich in antioxidants and vitamin C, which help combat oxidative stress and inflammation. Salmon is well known for its high content of omega-3 fatty acids, which are essential for reducing inflammation and supporting brain and heart health.

Understanding the importance of micronutrients, which include vitamins and minerals, is crucial for anyone looking to reduce inflammation and enhance their overall metabolic health. These tiny nutrients play significant roles in hundreds of body functions, from repairing cellular damage to supporting your immune system. They're essential for converting food into energy, repairing cellular damage, and bolstering your body's ability to recover and defend against environmental stressors. For instance, vitamin C supports your immune system and is a powerful antioxidant that helps reduce inflammation. Magnesium, another essential micronutrient, supports muscle and nerve function and helps maintain blood pressure levels, which can be beneficial in managing chronic inflammation.

Introducing superfoods into your diet is another fantastic way to increase nutrient density. Superfoods are typically rich in compounds that offer significant health benefits beyond their essential nutritional value. Take turmeric, for example, known for its curcumin content, which has potent anti-inflammatory properties.

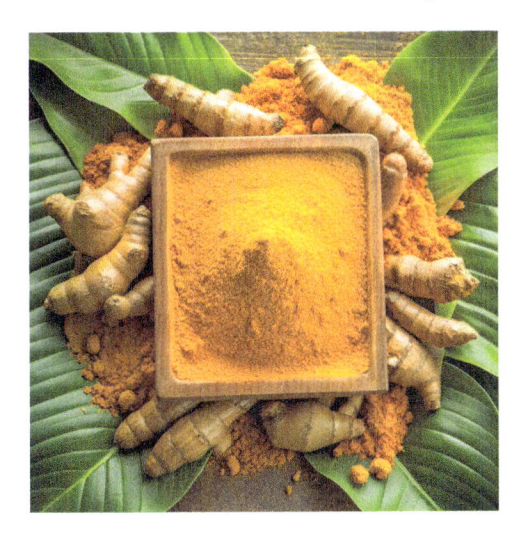

Incorporating turmeric into your diet can be as simple as adding a teaspoon to a smoothie or sprinkling it into a stir-fry, giving your meal an anti-inflammatory boost.

Green tea is another superfood rich in antioxidants called catechins, which reduce inflammation and support healthy cellular function. Then there's flaxseed, which delivers a healthy dose of fiber and omega-3 fatty acids known for their anti-inflammatory effects. Grinding flaxseeds and adding them to your yogurt, smoothies, or baked goods is an easy way to enhance the nutrient profile of your meals.

Consider some practical tips for incorporating these nutrient-dense foods into your everyday meals. A simple strategy is sprinkling seeds like flaxseeds or chia seeds onto salads or smoothies.

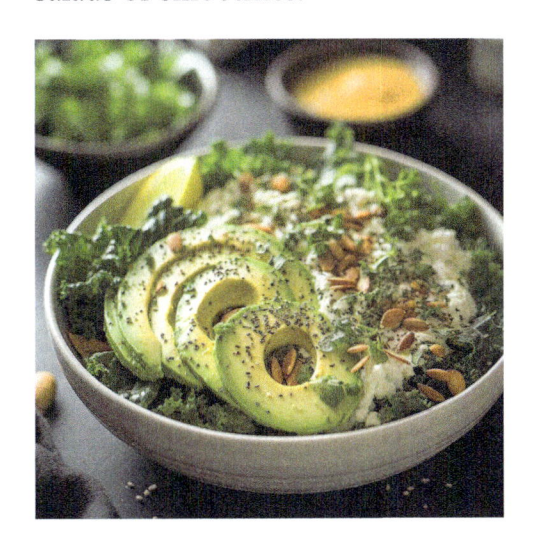

These seeds boost the nutrient content and add a pleasant crunch or thickness to your meals. Another tip is to use vegetable-based pasta alternatives, such as zucchini noodles or spaghetti squash, which can dramatically increase the nutrient density of a traditional pasta dish. Swapping out regular pasta for these alternatives adds more fiber and vitamins to your meal without sacrificing satisfaction or flavor. Moreover, make it a habit to incorporate at least one leafy green or brightly colored vegetable into every meal. Whether it's spinach in your morning omelet, a mixed berry salad for lunch, or roasted carrots and beets with dinner, these foods provide a spectrum of nutrients and antioxidants that support a healthy, anti-inflammatory diet.

By focusing on these nutrient-dense foods, you're not just filling your plate with delicious items but also significantly enhancing the quality of your diet. Every meal becomes an opportunity to nourish your body with the vital nutrients it needs to function at its best, reduce inflammation, and enhance your overall well-being. This approach to eating encourages not only a healthier lifestyle but also a more vibrant, energetic life.

TRACKING YOUR PROGRESS: TOOLS AND TECHNIQUES

Navigating an anti-inflammatory diet isn't just about making dietary changes; it's about making them stick. One of the most effective ways to do this is by keeping a food diary or using mobile apps designed to track your food intake, macronutrient breakdown, and caloric intake. Think of these tools as your personal diet assistants. They don't just record what you eat; they provide insights into your eating patterns, helping you understand where you might need to adjust. For instance, a food diary app can quickly show if you're consistently overdoing it on carbs but skimping on proteins or if your calorie intake is higher on weekends. This immediate feedback is invaluable, allowing you to see patterns you might otherwise miss and adjust accordingly.

These digital tools can also help you rigorously adhere to your anti-inflammatory diet. By recording your meals, you become more mindful of your eating. Are you incorporating enough anti-inflammatory foods like berries, nuts, and leafy greens? Are there days when processed foods creep in more than they should? A food diary holds you accountable and keeps your dietary goals top of mind, which can be especially helpful when you're just starting out and still finding your way around this new way of eating. Many apps also allow you to track your water intake, exercise, and even how you're feeling, giving you a holistic view of your health and how your diet impacts your overall well-being.

Another crucial element is setting realistic goals for managing your anti-inflammatory diet effectively. Goals give you a target to aim for and help motivate you to stick to your dietary changes. However, the key is to ensure these goals are achievable. If you're new to anti-inflammatory eating, a goal like "Incorporate a serving of leafy greens into every meal" is specific, measurable, and more manageable than a vague "Eat healthier." As you progress, these goals can evolve. After a month, you aim to have two meat-free days a week or replace all refined sugars with natural sweeteners. Adjusting your goals as you grow more accustomed to this way of eating keeps you challenged and prevents you from feeling overwhelmed.

Feedback loops and adjustments are integral to this process. Let's say you've set a goal to reduce your sugar intake. After a week, you review your food diary and notice that your sugar intake drops during the week but spikes on weekends. This insight allows you to strategize ways to address these spikes, perhaps by preparing healthier weekend snacks ahead of time or planning activities that don't center around sugary treats. These adjustments, informed by consistent tracking and reflection, help refine your diet and make your anti-inflammatory eating habits more effective and sustainable.

You might also feel stuck or need help further optimizing your diet. Involving a health professional, such as a dietitian or nutritionist, can be very beneficial at this stage.

These experts can analyze your food diary and provide tailored advice beyond general guidelines. They can help troubleshoot issues like persistent digestive discomfort or plateauing weight loss and suggest dietary tweaks informed by professional knowledge and experience. For instance, if you're struggling with ongoing inflammation despite making significant dietary changes, a nutritionist can help you identify potential food sensitivities or nutritional deficiencies that might contribute to the problem.

Incorporating these tools and techniques into your approach to an anti-inflammatory diet transforms it from a mere eating plan into a comprehensive lifestyle change. Tracking your progress, setting realistic goals, constantly adjusting based on feedback, and seeking professional advice are all strategies that enhance your ability to follow an anti-inflammatory diet and thrive on it. As you become more attuned to your body's responses and refine your dietary choices, you'll likely find that this way of eating becomes a natural part of your daily routine, seamlessly supporting your health and well-being.

OVERCOMING WEIGHT LOSS PLATEAUS

Hitting a weight loss plateau can feel like running into an invisible wall, and, honestly, it can be pretty frustrating. If you're sticking to your diet, exercising, and doing all the right things, the scales suddenly won't budge. What gives? Well, weight loss plateaus are a normal part of the weight loss process, often resulting from metabolic adaptations. As you lose weight, your body requires fewer calories to function than at a heavier weight. So, the calorie deficit initially causes your weight loss to decrease, and your metabolism might slow down to conserve energy, leading to a plateau.

To break through this plateau, consider shaking things up. Changing your exercise routine is a great start. If you've been jogging every morning, throw in weight training or a yoga class.

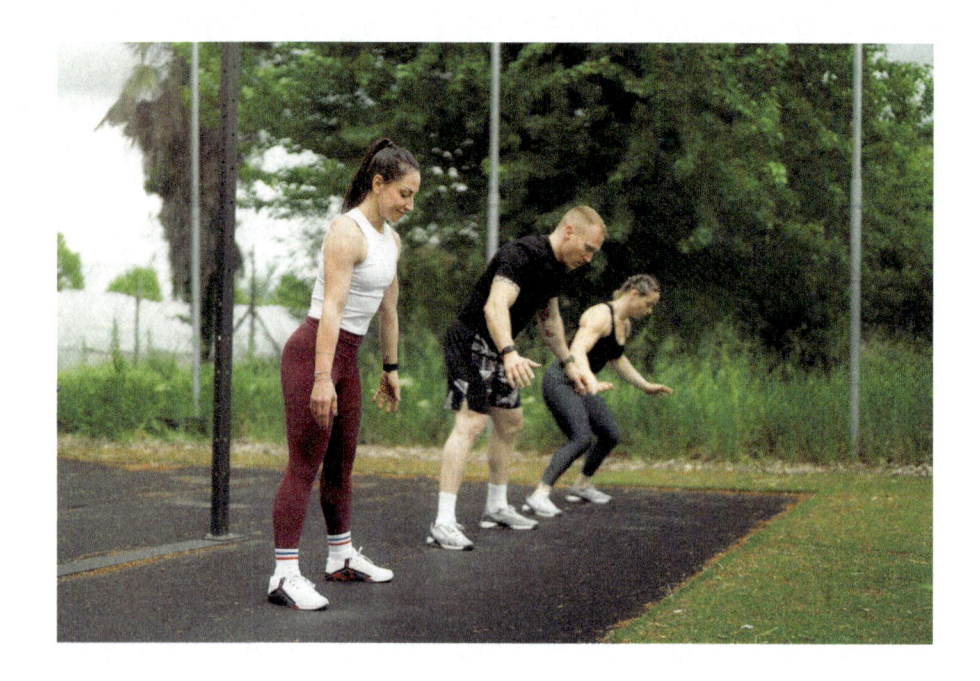

Different types of exercise challenge your body in new ways, which can jumpstart your metabolism. Adjusting your calorie intake can also help. As counterintuitive as it might sound, increasing your calories can reassure your body that it's not starvation; it's boosting your metabolism. Conversely, if you've become a bit lax with calorie tracking, tightening up your food diary might reveal hidden calories that are sneaking in.

Increasing your protein intake is another effective strategy. Protein can help prevent muscle loss, which is crucial because losing muscle mass can decrease your metabolic rate. Foods rich in protein can also increase the amount of energy your body expends digesting them, known as the thermic effect of food. Including a source of lean protein in every meal and snack can help you break through a plateau and support continued weight loss.

However, it's not just about what you do; it's also about how you think. The psychological aspects of encountering a plateau can sometimes be the most challenging. Feeling discouraged or losing focus is easy when you don't see the expected results. Setting small, achievable goals can help maintain your motivation. Instead of focusing solely on the scale, celebrate other signs of progress, such as feeling more energetic, sleeping better, or your clothes fitting more comfortably. These victories can provide a much-needed morale boost.

Maintaining a long-term perspective is crucial. Weight management is not just a phase but a permanent lifestyle change. Patience and persistence are your best friends on this journey. Continually reassessing your goals and strategies, adjusting as needed, and staying committed to your plan will eventually help you overcome plateaus. Remember, it's not about how quickly you reach your destination but about finding sustainable habits you can stick with for life.

As this chapter closes, remember that managing weight and maintaining a healthy lifestyle requires a balance of knowledge, strategies, and patience. You've learned how to address a weight loss plateau, understand the complex dance of calories and macronutrients, and understand the importance of incorporating nutrient-dense foods into your diet. This foundation will help you manage your weight and enhance your overall health. As we move forward, in the next chapter we will explore understanding and managing common health conditions with dietary adjustments, providing deeper insights and practical tips to address specific health challenges through diet. With this understanding, you can customize your eating habits to your particular nutritional needs, further improving the benefits of your anti-inflammatory lifestyle.

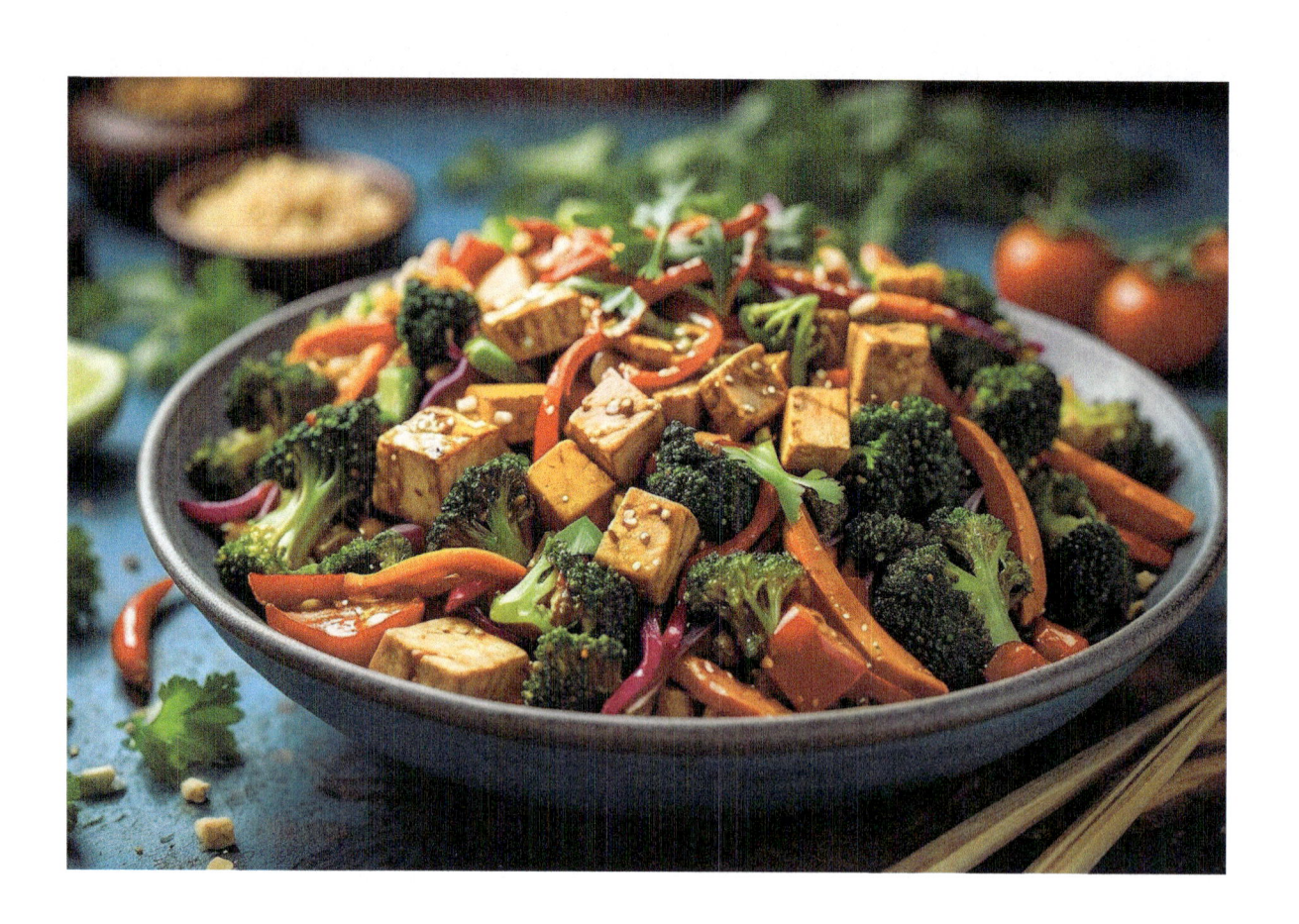

4

SPECIAL DIETARY CONSIDERATIONS AND SUBSTITUTIONS

Navigating the world of food allergies, sensitivities, and personal dietary needs can sometimes feel like trying to solve a complex puzzle. Each piece represents a different aspect of your diet, and finding out where each one fits can be a journey of discovery. This chapter guides you through making informed choices about what to eat, especially if you must avoid certain ingredients like gluten. Whether dealing with specific health concerns or just aiming to feel your best, understanding how to adjust your diet to meet your body's needs is empowering and can set you on a path to improved well-being.

GLUTEN-FREE ANTI-INFLAMMATORY EATING

Identifying Gluten Sources

Gluten can hide in products beyond the obvious bread and pastries, including sauces, soups, and condiments like soy sauce. Learning to identify these hidden sources is like becoming a dietary detective, examining labels, and understanding the terminology that can indicate the presence of gluten. For instance, terms like "malt" (derived from barley) and "seitan" (a wheat-based protein) are critical indicators of gluten. This detective work is crucial not only for those with celiac disease but also for anyone looking to reduce inflammation through diet, as gluten can irritate the gut and contribute to inflammatory responses.

Gluten-Free Grains

If you're avoiding gluten, you might worry about missing out on a whole range of foods, but there's a world of gluten-free grains that are both delicious and nutritious. Quinoa, for example, is an excellent gluten-free option and a complete protein since it has all nine essential amino acids. Despite its name, buckwheat is another gluten-free powerhouse rich in fiber and antioxidants. Millet's mild flavor and versatility are excellent in everything from breakfast porridges to dinner side dishes. Incorporating these grains into your meals can boost your nutritional intake, diversifying your diet in delicious and health-supportive ways.

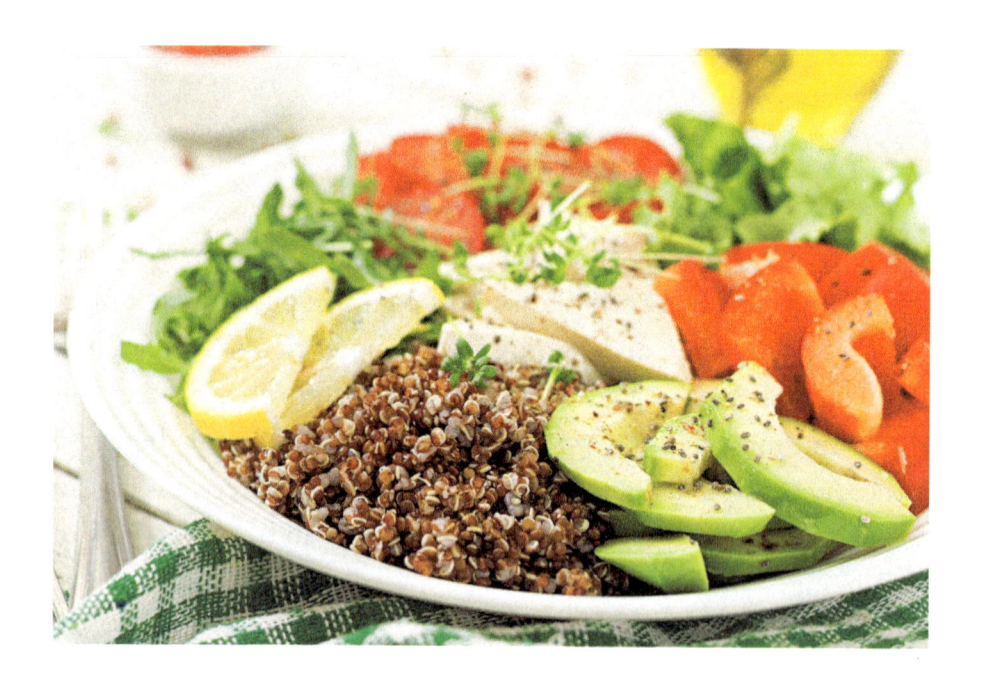

Cross-Contamination Concerns

As important as avoiding gluten is for people with extreme gluten sensitivity or celiac disease, so is avoiding cross-contamination. Having separate cooking and prep areas, utensils, and storage for gluten-free foods in the kitchen is crucial. It's like setting up a little gluten-free zone in your kitchen. Always wash cooking tools and surfaces thoroughly before preparing gluten-free meals, and consider having a dedicated toaster and other appliances if your sensitivity is severe. These steps help ensure that your efforts to avoid gluten are practical, keeping your meals safe and enjoyable without worrying about accidental exposure.

Gluten-Free Baking Tips

Baking gluten-free can initially seem daunting, but you can recreate all your favorite baked goods with a few tips and the right ingredients. Gluten-free baking often involves a mix of flour substitutes such as almond flour, rice flour, and potato starch. Each of these brings different qualities to your baked goods, affecting texture and flavor. For instance, almond flour adds moistness and a rich, nutty flavor, making it excellent for cakes and muffins. On the other hand, rice flour is great for achieving a light and fluffy texture in bread and cookies. Mixing several different flours to balance their qualities often yields the best results.

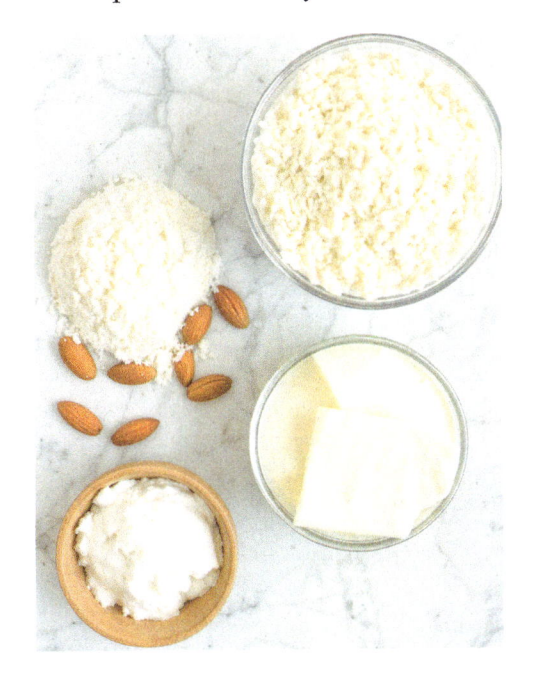

Remember, xanthan gum or guar gum is usually needed to replace the binding qualities of gluten. Start with small batches to test ratios, and don't be afraid to experiment—gluten-free baking is an art, and every attempt brings you closer to perfection.

As we explore these dietary adjustments and substitutions, remember that each change you make is a step toward a healthier, more vibrant you. Whether navigating gluten sensitivities, exploring new grains, or mastering the art of gluten-free baking, each choice and modification is integral to crafting a diet that supports your physical health and your enjoyment and satisfaction of eating. Embrace the process, enjoy the discoveries, and celebrate each meal as an opportunity to nourish and care for your body in the most delicious way possible.

DAIRY SUBSCRIPTIONS IN YOUR ANTI-INFLAMMATORY DIET

Navigating the dairy world can be tricky, especially when trying to reduce inflammation. For some, dairy is a nonissue, but for others, it can be a source of discomfort and inflammation, particularly if you're lactose intolerant or have a dairy sensitivity. Understanding this connection is critical to managing your dietary needs effectively. Dairy products, including milk, cheese, and yogurt, can lead to inflammatory responses in some individuals, primarily due to lactose, the sugar in milk. For those who are lactose intolerant, the inability of the body to break down lactose results in gastrointestinal symptoms such as gas, bloating, and discomfort. But it's not just the lactose; specific proteins in dairy, like casein and whey, can also trigger inflammation, especially in people who are sensitive or allergic to them.

Transitioning to dairy-free alternatives can be a breath of fresh air if you've struggled with these issues. The good news is that the variety of nondairy milks available today is more extensive and accessible than ever. Almond milk, for example, is a popular choice known for its light, nutty flavor, making it a great addition to cereals, smoothies, and coffee.

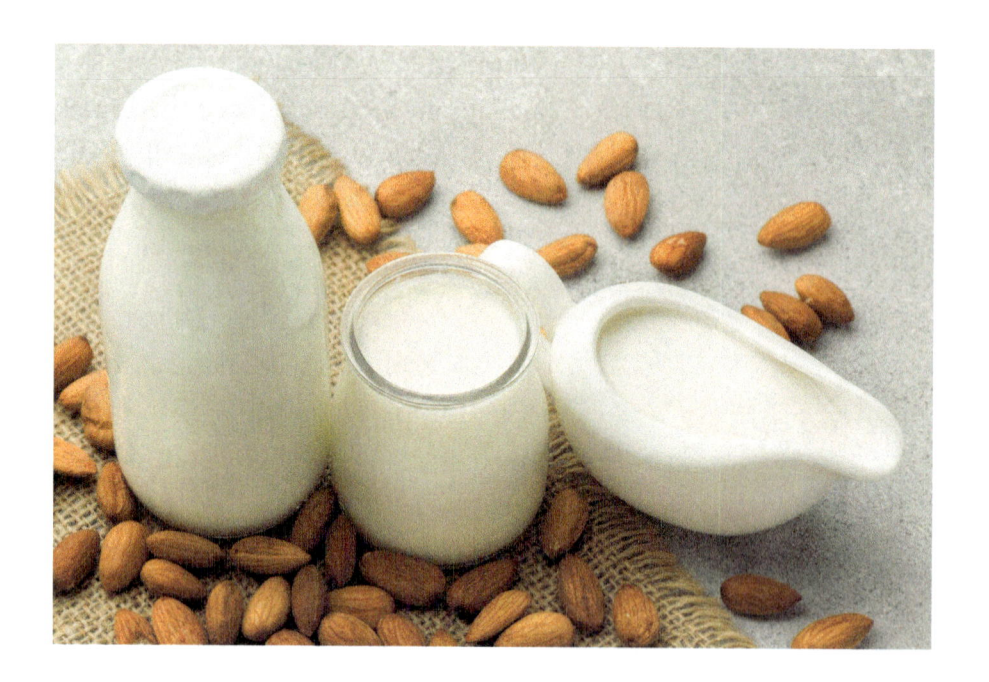

It's low in calories and, if fortified, can be a good source of calcium. However, almond milk might not be for you if you're allergic to nuts. In that case, oat milk could be an excellent alternative. Rich and slightly sweet, oat milk is fantastic for baked goods and pancakes, giving them a lovely texture and flavor. It's also high in fiber and beta-glucans, known for their cholesterol-lowering effects. Then there's coconut milk, which stands out with its creamy texture and tropical flavor. It's great in soups, curries, and desserts and is lactose-free, making it suitable for those with lactose intolerance. Each option has its own unique nutritional profile and uses in cooking and baking, so you might use a combination of both, depending on your culinary needs.

SPECIAL DIETARY CONSIDERATIONS AND SUBSTITUTIONS | 55

Let's remember that cheese and yogurt are staples in many diets but also potential sources of inflammation for some. The good news is that the range of plant-based cheese and yogurt alternatives has grown significantly, offering delicious and healthier substitutions. When choosing these products, it's essential to read the labels carefully. Look for options free of unnecessary additives and preservatives, which can also trigger inflammatory responses. Many plant-based cheeses come from nuts like cashews, which provide a creamy texture and are often seasoned with nutritional yeast to give a cheesy flavor without the dairy. Plant-based yogurts made from coconut, almonds, or oats can be a delightful part of your breakfast or snack routine, often containing live probiotic cultures beneficial for your gut health.

If you're feeling adventurous, making your dairy substitutes at home can be a rewarding experience. Homemade nut milks are surprisingly simple to make and allow you to control what goes into them exactly—no additives or sweeteners unless you add them.

Almonds are soaked for a whole night, blended with water, and then strained.

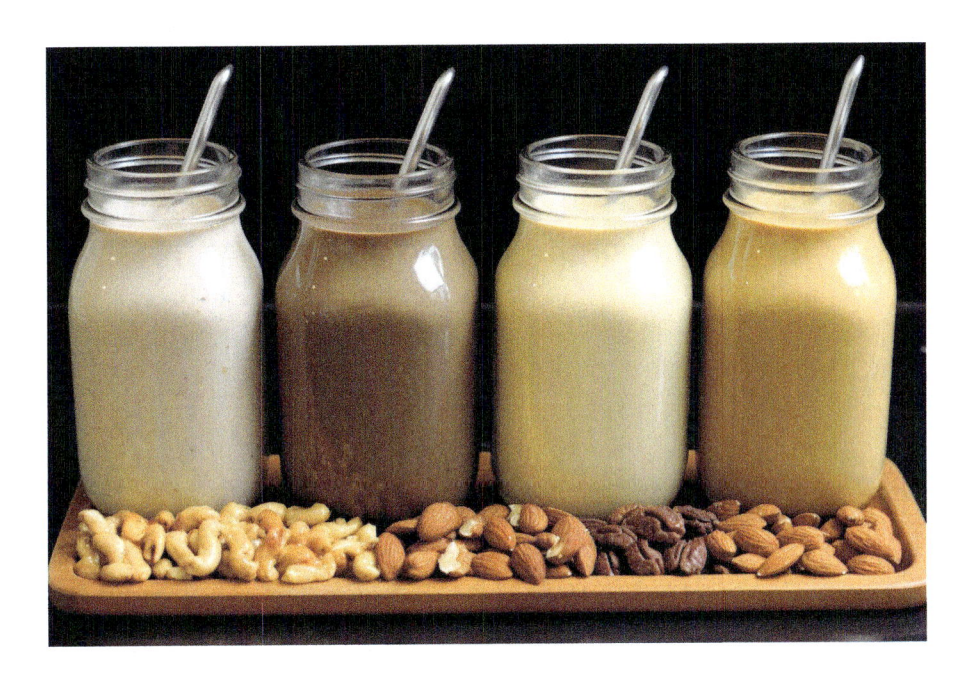

You are providing fresh, clean-tasting almond milk. Cashew cheese is another easy homemade alternative, requiring just soaked cashews, nutritional yeast, lemon juice, garlic, and some seasonings blended until smooth. These homemade options reduce your intake of processed foods and give you the satisfaction of knowing what you're eating, all while keeping inflammation in check.

Embracing dairy-free alternatives doesn't mean sacrificing flavor or variety in your diet. Whether using store-bought options or making your own, the world of nondairy substitutes offers a rich palette of flavors and textures. Making this change can lead to noticeable improvements in how you feel, mainly if dairy has caused you discomfort in the past. As you experiment with these substitutions, they open up new culinary possibilities, transforming your meals and health in the most delicious ways.

VEGETARIAN AND VEGAN OPTIONS FOR EVERY MEAL

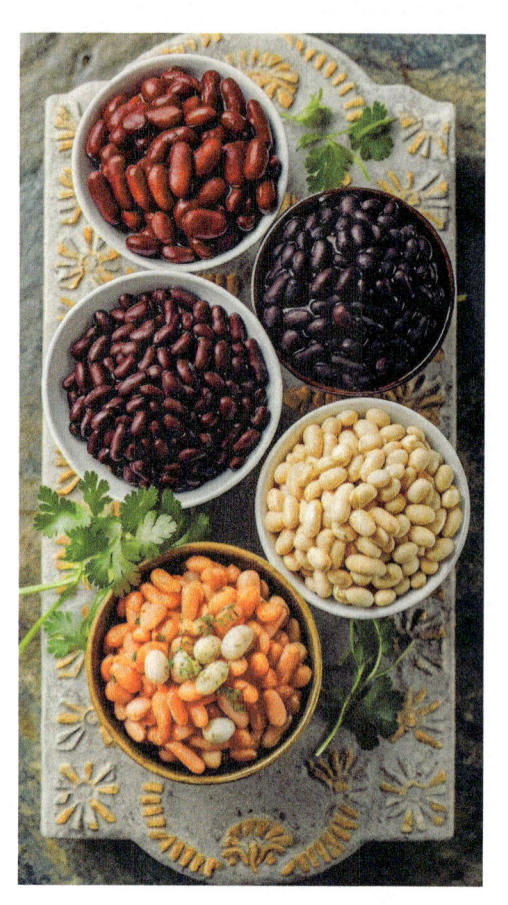

One common concern might be getting enough protein when embracing a vegetarian or vegan lifestyle. Your body needs protein as an essential building block for numerous functions, including the production of enzymes and the repair of muscles. Fortunately, plant-based diets offer a rich array of protein sources that are not only diverse but also packed with additional health benefits. Legumes, such as lentils, chickpeas, and black beans, are fantastic protein-rich foods that provide fiber, iron, and B vitamins. Incorporating these into your meals can boost your protein intake while supporting your body's overall health. For a twist, try using chickpeas in salads or homemade veggie burgers.

Lentils work beautifully in soups and stews, which are comforting and nutritious, especially during the cooler months. Then there are the complete proteins, or all of the necessary amino acids your body needs, found in soybeans, which are the source of the protein powerhouses tofu and tempeh.

Tofu is incredibly versatile, absorbing flavors from other ingredients, making it perfect for various dishes, from stir-fries to smoothies. Tempeh, conversely, has a nuttier flavor and a firmer texture, making it excellent for grilling or adding to sandwiches. Both are high in calcium and iron, needed for healthy bones and blood oxygen transport. They are also beneficial for protein intake. However, it's not just about protein. A balanced diet of other vital elements, such as iron, zinc, and vitamin B12, which are frequently found in large amounts in animal products, is necessary. The production of hemoglobin, a protein found in red blood cells that transports oxygen throughout the body, requires iron. Good plant sources include lentils, chickpeas, and cooked spinach. Pair these foods with vitamin C-rich items like tomatoes or citrus fruits to enhance iron absorption. Zinc is essential for immune function and cell growth, with pumpkin seeds and cashews being excellent plant-based sources. Vitamin B12, vital for nerve function and DNA and red blood cell production, can be more challenging in a plant-based diet. Nutritional yeast, fortified cereals, and plant-based milks are good options to include in your meals.

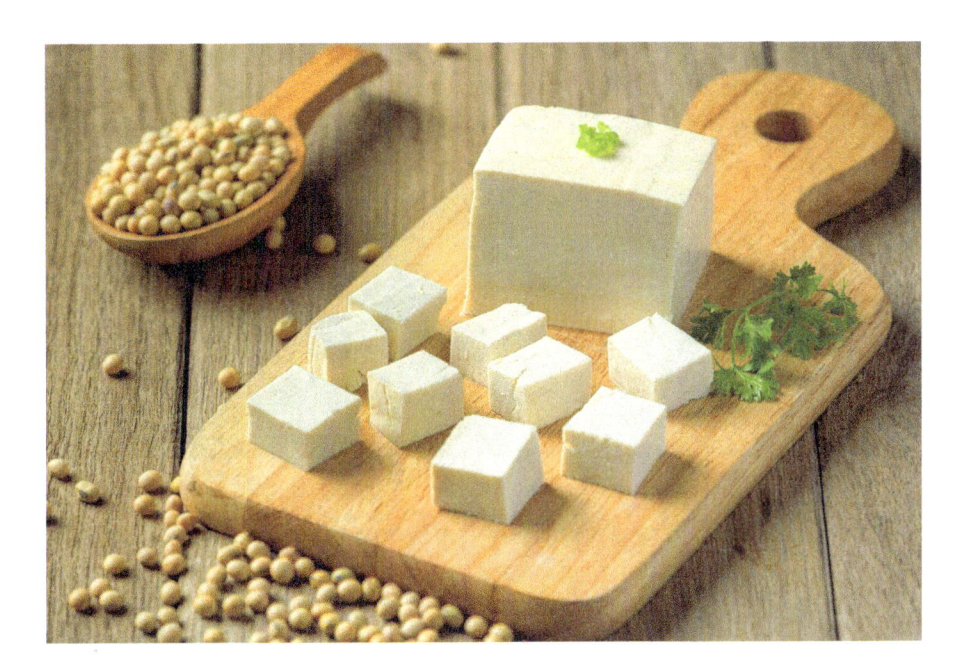

Incorporating various foods into your diet ensures you get a broad spectrum of nutrients and keeps your meals exciting and flavorful. Experiment with different beans, seeds, and greens to discover new favorite dishes that keep you satisfied and healthy. For instance, start your day with a smoothie bowl topped with a sprinkle of chia seeds, hemp seeds, and a dollop of almond butter—all superior sources of omega-3 fatty acids and protein. A quinoa salad with mixed beans, vibrant peppers, and a lemon-tahini dressing can be filling and refreshing for lunch. Dinner might feature a hearty vegetable and lentil stew enriched with iron-packed kale and served with whole-grain bread.

Consider this sample meal plan to illustrate the potential of a vegetarian or vegan diet. Breakfast could be a tofu scramble with spinach, mushrooms, and tomatoes, spiced with turmeric and black pepper for added anti-inflammatory benefits. A midmorning snack might include a small bowl of mixed nuts and dried fruits, providing a quick energy boost and a source of healthy fats. Lunch could be a vibrant Buddha bowl with a base of brown rice, topped with steamed broccoli, roasted sweet potatoes, and a generous helping of chickpeas, drizzled with an avocado lime dressing.

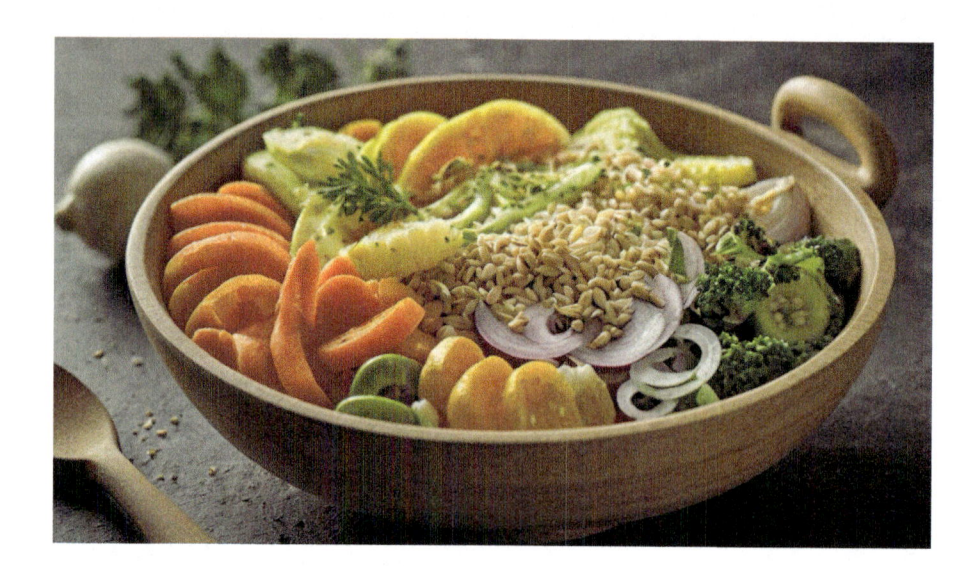

Carrot sticks with hummus are a crunchy, satisfying option for an afternoon snack. Dinner could then be a tempeh stir-fry with various colorful vegetables and a side of quinoa, ensuring a filling end to your day with a balance of protein, fiber, and essential nutrients.

This type of meal planning ensures that you meet your nutritional needs and aligns with anti-inflammatory eating principles. It provides a wide range of antioxidants and other health-promoting compounds in plant foods. These meals showcase the diversity available within a plant-based diet, proving that choosing to eat vegetarian or vegan doesn't mean sacrificing flavor or nutrition. Instead, it opens up a world of colorful, creative, and healthful eating options that benefit your body and the planet.

NUT-FREE SNACKS AND MEALS FOR ALLERGY SUFFERERS

Understanding safe snacking options and meal choices becomes crucial when managing nut allergies, whether for yourself or a family member. Navigating this can feel like setting up a safety net that ensures everyone can eat without worry. Let's explore some nut-free snacks that are safe, delicious, and nutritious. Snacking on fruits and vegetables is always a great choice. You can dip carrot sticks, cucumber slices, or apple wedges in nut-free butter like sunflower butter, which offers a creamy texture and a pleasant, mild taste similar to peanut butter but without allergens. Sunflower or even pumpkin seeds make for a crunchy snack packed with nutrients like magnesium, which helps with muscle and nerve function, and zinc, which is vital for immune health.

Another fantastic option is homemade popcorn tossed with olive oil, sea salt, or nutritional yeast for a cheesy flavor. It's whole grain, high in fiber, and surprisingly filling, making it perfect for movie nights or on-the-go snacks. For those with a sweet tooth, rice cakes topped with coconut yogurt and fresh berries offer a delightful treat that's easy to prepare and satisfying. These snacks keep you full between meals and support an anti-inflammatory diet with their range of vitamins, minerals, and antioxidants.

Reading food labels is another critical skill you'll want to develop. It's about more than just checking for nut ingredients; it's about understanding the potential for cross-contamination and the signs that a product might not be safe. Look for labels that mention if the product was made in a facility that processes nuts, as this can pose a risk for those with severe allergies. Familiarize yourself with the names under which nuts can be listed, such as almonds, hazelnuts, or walnuts. Be wary of vague terms like "natural flavors" or "spices," which can sometimes include nut products. This vigilance ensures you can choose safe snacks and ingredients, keeping allergic reactions at bay.

Many alternatives exist for those who need to steer clear of nuts but still want to ensure adequate protein intake. Legumes such as chickpeas, lentils, and beans are fantastic protein sources and are entirely nut-free.

You can turn them into delicious dishes like hummus (using tahini as a sesame-based alternative to nut butter), lentil salads, or bean chili. These foods not only provide the needed protein but are also high in fiber and low in fat, supporting overall health and helping to manage inflammation. Quinoa and chia seeds are excellent protein sources and versatile enough for various dishes, from breakfast porridge to dinner entrees. Creating a nut-free environment at home, especially in households with allergic children, starts with educating all family members about allergies and avoiding cross-contamination. Establish designated areas in your kitchen for preparing and storing nut-free foods, and have separate utensils and cooking equipment. Regularly cleaning surfaces and storing nut-containing products securely and separately can reduce exposure risk. Regardless of dietary limitations, these acts establish an ideal eating atmosphere, comforting everyone and enabling them to share meals without worrying about adverse reactions.

Homemade nut milks are surprisingly simple to make and allow you to control what goes into them exactly—no additives or sweeteners unless you add them. You can create an enjoyable eating environment that supports your health goals and dietary needs by choosing safe, nutritious snacks and meals, understanding how to read labels effectively, and ensuring your kitchen is set up to avoid cross-contamination. As you continue exploring and adapting these strategies, you'll find that managing a nut-free diet is feasible and rewarding, allowing you and your loved ones to eat confidently and enjoyably.

LOW-FODMAP CHOICES FOR SENSITIVE STOMACHS

If you've ever experienced the discomfort of a bloated, painful stomach without an apparent reason, the culprit might be lurking in your daily meals under the guise of FODMAPs. FODMAPs, which stands for Fermentable Oligosaccharides, Disaccharides, Monosaccharides, and Polyols, are carbohydrates that are not easily absorbed by the gut. Certain undigested carbohydrates can cause discomfort for some people as they move through the digestive tract, where gut bacteria ferment them, leading to gas, bloating, and pain. Individuals with irritable bowel syndrome (IBS) or similar gastrointestinal sensitivities are significantly affected. Understanding FODMAPs is the first step in managing these symptoms effectively, allowing you to enjoy your meals without the dread of discomfort.

Navigating which foods are high and low in FODMAPs is essential for this dietary adjustment. High-FODMAP foods include onions, garlic, certain legumes, wheat-based products, and some fruits such as apples and pears. Dairy products that contain lactose can also be problematic for those sensitive to FODMAPs. On the other hand, many foods are considered low-FODMAP and can help keep your stomach calm. These include leafy greens, carrots, cucumbers, oranges, strawberries, and proteins like eggs, tofu, and most seafood. Another good option is a grain, like rice, quinoa, or oats. You can significantly reduce the symptoms of IBS and associated disorders by concentrating your diet on low-FODMAP foods. Incorporating low-FODMAP foods into an anti-inflammatory diet can seem challenging initially but is manageable with some planning and creativity. For instance, instead of using onion and garlic in your cooking—which are primary triggers for many with sensitive stomachs—try infusing your oils with these flavors. Sauté garlic or onions in oil, then remove them and use the infused oil to flavor your dishes without the FODMAPs. Herbs like basil, chives, oregano, and spices like turmeric and ginger are low in FODMAPs and possess potent anti-inflammatory properties, making them excellent additions to your meals. Furthermore, embracing a variety of colorful vegetables and fruits that are low in FODMAPs ensures you're still getting a spectrum of antioxidants and phytochemicals crucial for combating inflammation.

The journey to a low-FODMAP diet is highly personal and involves a phase of adjustment and experimentation. It typically starts with a strict elimination of all high-FODMAP foods. This period allows your digestive system to settle and your symptoms to subside. After this phase, you can begin reintroducing foods one at a time, monitoring how your body responds to each. This process helps you identify specific foods that trigger symptoms, allowing you to create a personalized eating plan that keeps your symptoms at bay. Keep a food diary during this phase; it can be invaluable in tracking which foods cause issues and how to adjust your diet to minimize discomfort.

Balancing a low-FODMAP diet with anti-inflammatory eating principles might seem like a tightrope walk, but it's achievable with some knowledge and preparation. Planning meals around low-FODMAP and anti-inflammatory foods can open up a new world of culinary possibilities, transforming your diet into one that supports your digestive health while also helping reduce inflammation. Whether whipping up a smoothie with low-FODMAP fruits like oranges and strawberries or creating a hearty salad with greens and an array of colorful veggies, the key is to focus on what you can eat rather than what you can't. With each meal, you're feeding your body and nurturing it, giving it the tools it needs to heal and thrive. This approach eases your digestive symptoms and enhances your overall health, making every meal a step toward a happier, healthier you.

ADAPTING RECIPES FOR THE WHOLE FAMILY

When it comes to feeding a family, especially on an anti-inflammatory diet, the trick is not just in choosing the right ingredients but also in making sure the meals appeal to everyone, from the pickiest toddlers to the most health-conscious adults. Adapting your family meals to be delicious and anti-inflammatory is a balancing act. Still, with a few creative strategies, you can satisfy various taste preferences and dietary needs without turning into a short-order cook.

One practical approach is to prepare base meals that you can easily customize. Imagine making a stir-fry for dinner; you can cook a big batch of veggies and a simple protein like grilled chicken. Then, serve it with different add-ons and sides, like brown rice, quinoa, or spiralized zucchini noodles. Each family member can pick the base and toppings that suit their taste or dietary restrictions. This method saves you from preparing multiple meals and encourages family members to experiment with new flavors and ingredients, gradually expanding their nutritional preferences.

Involving your family in the meal preparation process can also be a game-changer. When kids and partners participate in cooking, they're more likely to eat what they've made. Start simple: Let younger children wash veggies or mix salad dressings, while older kids and adults might chop vegetables or manage the stovetop with supervision. With these activities, preparing meals becomes a fun family activity and a great chance to talk about the health advantages of your ingredients. Explain why you're using olive oil over butter or choosing whole grains instead of white flour and how these choices help reduce inflammation and support overall health.

Moreover, using mealtime as an educational opportunity can benefit your family's dietary habits. Discuss why certain foods are part of your anti-inflammatory diet and their specific benefits, such as how omega-3 fatty acids in salmon can help reduce joint pain or how berries high in antioxidants can aid muscle recovery and repair. This knowledge helps build a positive connection between the foods we eat and how we feel, making healthy eating more appealing and impactful.

Lastly, remember that dietary changes, especially significant ones like shifting to an anti-inflammatory diet, can take time to adjust. Be patient and open to feedback from your family members. Their participation in choosing and preparing meals can lead to more sustainable and enjoyable dietary habits, fostering a healthier lifestyle for everyone involved.

As you continue to explore and adapt these strategies, remember that each meal is an opportunity to nourish the body and the family bond. You transform mealtime into a nurturing experience that extends well beyond the kitchen by cooking, learning, and eating together. These moments of connection and care make the dietary transition manageable and deeply rewarding.

Summarizing the essence of this chapter, we've navigated through adapting family meals to an anti-inflammatory diet, involving everyone in the cooking process, and using mealtime as an educational moment. These strategies aim to make healthy eating a shared commitment and a delightful part of your family's life. As we move forward, we'll delve deeper into understanding specific anti-inflammatory nutrients and how to incorporate them into your daily meals, ensuring that every dish brings pleasure and health benefits.

YOUR FEEDBACK CAN CHANGE LIVES

Would you help someone you've never met, even if you never got credit for it?

This is your chance to make a difference for someone struggling with inflammation and searching for guidance. Your review can inspire them to take the first step toward better health.

It's simple:

📱 Scan the QR code below.

💬 Leave your review in less than 60 seconds.

https://www.amazon.com/review/create-review/?asin=B0DQDZYSLZ

Your input could inspire healthier living, improve well-being, and empower someone to take control of their health journey.

Thank you for spreading kindness and helping us make the anti-inflammatory lifestyle accessible to all!

Your biggest fan,

— Lynn Benedetto

PS: If you know someone who could benefit from this book, please share it with them.

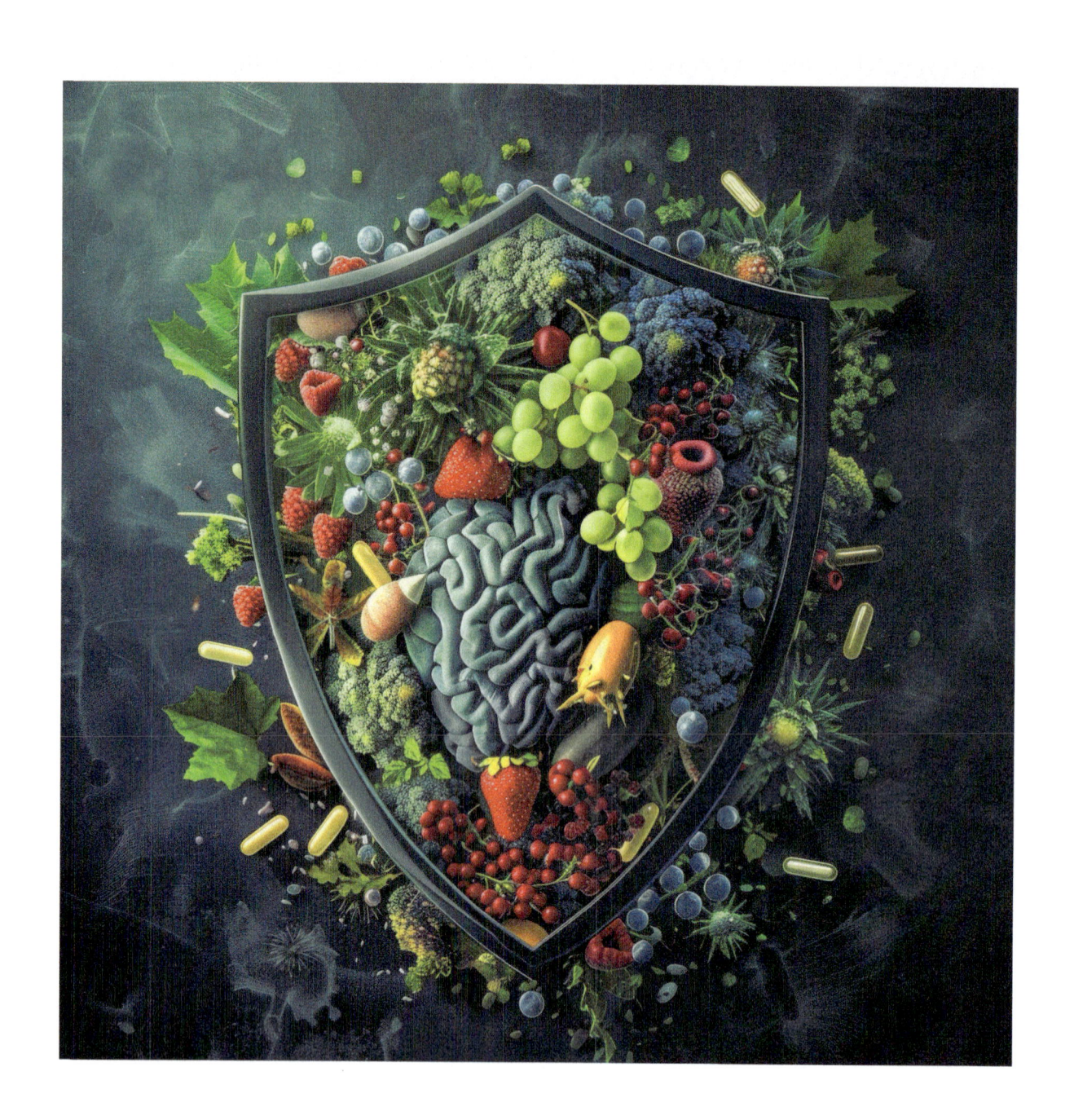

5

ENHANCING GUT HEALTH AND IMMUNITY

Imagine your gut as a bustling city with trillions of residents—bacteria, fungi, and viruses—each with a crucial role in how your body functions. This bustling metropolis isn't just about digestion; it's central to your overall health, influencing everything from your immune system to your mood. Understanding how to keep this vital city thriving will boost your digestion and enhance your mental clarity and resilience against diseases. Let's dive into the fascinating world of your gut microbiome, uncovering how a balanced digestive system can transform your health from the inside out.

THE GUT-HEALTH CONNECTION: BASICS YOU NEED TO KNOW

Introduction to the Gut Microbiome

Your gut microbiome is like a complex ecosystem, hosting diverse organisms that play different roles in your health. These microorganisms, primarily bacteria, are involved in numerous critical processes, including digesting the food you eat, absorbing nutrients, and even manufacturing vitamins B and K, which are crucial for blood clotting and energy production. But their influence doesn't stop there. The balance of these microbial communities also affects how your immune system functions, how your body responds to infections, and how efficiently you can fend off diseases. Keeping this community in balance means feeding it what it needs—lots of fiber, minimal sugars, and a variety of nutrients—while protecting it from what can cause disruptions, like excessive antibiotics or a diet high in processed foods. It's like keeping the city's infrastructure in top shape to ensure everything runs smoothly.

Gut as the Second Brain

Have you ever had a "gut feeling" about something? This isn't just a metaphor. The gut-brain axis is a communication network linking your gut and brain, physically through nerves and chemically through hormones and neurotransmitters. This connection means that the state of your gut can directly influence your mental health, affecting everything from your mood to your ability to handle stress. For instance, the gut produces a significant portion of the body's serotonin, the feel-good neurotransmitter. An imbalance in your gut flora can contribute to feelings of depression or anxiety. This connection highlights the importance of maintaining a healthy gut microbiome for overall mental wellbeing. Exploring dietary changes and consulting with healthcare professionals can provide strategies to support gut health and improve mental health. Nurturing your gut health can thus not only keep your digestive system happy but elevate your mental well-being.

Barrier Function of the Gut

Your gut has another crucial role: acting as a barrier that protects your body from external pathogens. Think of it as the city walls that keep invaders at bay. This barrier function is crucial in preventing substances from leaking into the rest of your body and triggering immune responses, a condition often called "leaky gut" syndrome. When the gut's lining is compromised, unwanted substances like toxins and undigested food particles can escape into your bloodstream, leading to inflammation and potentially contributing to various issues, including allergies, autoimmune diseases, and chronic inflammatory conditions. Maintaining a robust and intact gut lining is, therefore, paramount. Focus on your diet and ensure you consume enough nutrients like zinc and amino acids to help repair and maintain the gut wall.

Influence of Diet on Gut Health

Diet plays a pivotal role in the composition and health of your gut microbiome. What you eat can promote the growth of beneficial or harmful bacteria, tipping the balance of this delicate ecosystem. High-fiber foods, such as legumes, whole grains, and vegetables, fuel good bacteria, helping them thrive and function effectively. On the other hand, a diet high in sugars and fats can encourage the growth of bacteria that contribute to poor health outcomes. Fermented foods like yogurt, kefir, and sauerkraut are particularly beneficial as they introduce live probiotics into the gut, helping to enhance its diversity and functionality. Choosing your foods wisely directly impacts your overall health by nourishing the beneficial "residents" in your gut city.

Understanding your gut's health and its broad-reaching effects on your body is the first step in harnessing its power to enhance your overall well-being. By nurturing your gut through appropriate dietary choices and lifestyle habits, you're improving your digestion and setting the stage for better health across multiple body systems. It's a foundational aspect of your health that can yield tremendous benefits when cared for properly, echoing every aspect of your life.

PROBIOTICS AND PREBIOTICS: ALLIES IN YOUR ANTI-INFLAMMATORY DIET

Imagine walking through a garden where each plant helps the others thrive. Probiotics and prebiotics similarly work in your gut. Probiotics are live, beneficial bacteria that settle in your digestive system and help it function optimally. They are like the plants in our garden analogy—living organisms that can provide tremendous health benefits. On the other hand, prebiotics are the water and fertilizer that help these beneficial bacteria flourish. They are fibers and compounds that your body doesn't digest; instead, they serve as food for probiotics and support the growth of healthy bacteria in your gut.

Now, why is this important? The balance of bacteria in your gut affects not just digestion but your overall health, including your immune system, weight, and even mood. Mixing probiotic and prebiotic-rich foods can help maintain this balance, ensuring your gut works like a well-oiled machine. For probiotics, think of fermented foods that encourage good bacteria growth. These include yogurt, kefir, sauerkraut, and kimchi. When choosing yogurt or kefir, opt for versions that are low in sugar and have "live and active cultures" listed on the label. This substantial amount of beneficial bacteria indicates their effectiveness. Sauerkraut and kimchi, being probiotic-rich, are also packed with enzymes and vitamins that boost digestion and nutrient absorption.

Prebiotics are found in many vegetables, fruits, and whole grains. Foods like garlic, onions, bananas, and oats are excellent sources. These foods contain fibers and natural sugars like inulin and oligofructose that nurture gut bacteria. Imagine eating a bowl of oatmeal with banana slices—a filling breakfast and a meal feeding your microbiome, enhancing digestion and nutrient uptake.

Benefits of Gut Health and Beyond

The benefits of consuming a balanced amount of probiotics and prebiotics extend far beyond digestion. First and foremost, they help enhance your digestion, which allows for better nutrient absorption and less gastrointestinal discomfort. This can mean fewer episodes of bloating, gas, and irregular bowel movements. But the perks don't stop there. By strengthening your gut flora, you're also enhancing your immune system. A robust gut microbiome can help your body fend off infections more effectively and modulate your immune response, reducing chronic inflammation. Chronic inflammation's link to numerous health issues, including heart disease and diabetes, makes addressing it crucial.

Moreover, research has shown that the gut microbiome profoundly impacts health through the gut-brain axis. A healthy gut can contribute to better mood regulation and may decrease the risk of disorders like depression and anxiety. So, by nurturing your gut with probiotics and prebiotics, you're taking care of your physical and mental health.

Incorporating into the Daily Diet

Incorporating probiotics and prebiotics into your diet doesn't have to be complicated. A straightforward way is to start your day with a probiotic-rich yogurt or kefir. Adding a banana or a sprinkle of prebiotic-rich oats or flaxseeds can make it even more beneficial, enhancing the probiotic effect and keeping you full longer. For lunch or dinner, adding a side of sauerkraut or kimchi can boost your meal's flavor and probiotic content. Alternatively, consider cooking with garlic and onions more frequently. These can be sautéed as a base for soups, sauces, and stews, adding flavor and prebiotic power.

ENHANCING GUT HEALTH AND IMMUNITY | 71

Another enjoyable way to get your prebiotics is through snacks. A simple banana or oat-based granola bar can quickly boost prebiotics. Meanwhile, consider sipping on kefir or adding it to your smoothies for a probiotic punch. These quickly boost prebiotics to improve gut health and overall well-being significantly.

Understanding and embracing the roles of probiotics and prebiotics in your diet sets the stage for a healthier gut, which can lead to a healthier you. Remember, it's about creating a balance that supports your body, enhancing your health from the inside out. With these tools in your dietary arsenal, you're well on your way to nurturing your body's needs and ensuring your digestive system is functioning and thriving.

FOODS THAT BOOST YOUR IMMUNE SYSTEM NATURALLY

When you think about your immune system, imagine it as your body's security team, always on alert to defend you against invaders like bacteria and viruses. Like any dedicated team, it needs the proper support to function at its best. That's where your diet comes into play. Feeding your body specific nutrients can boost your immune system, helping it reduce illnesses more effectively. Let's explore some of these immune-boosting nutrients and how you can incorporate them into your meals.

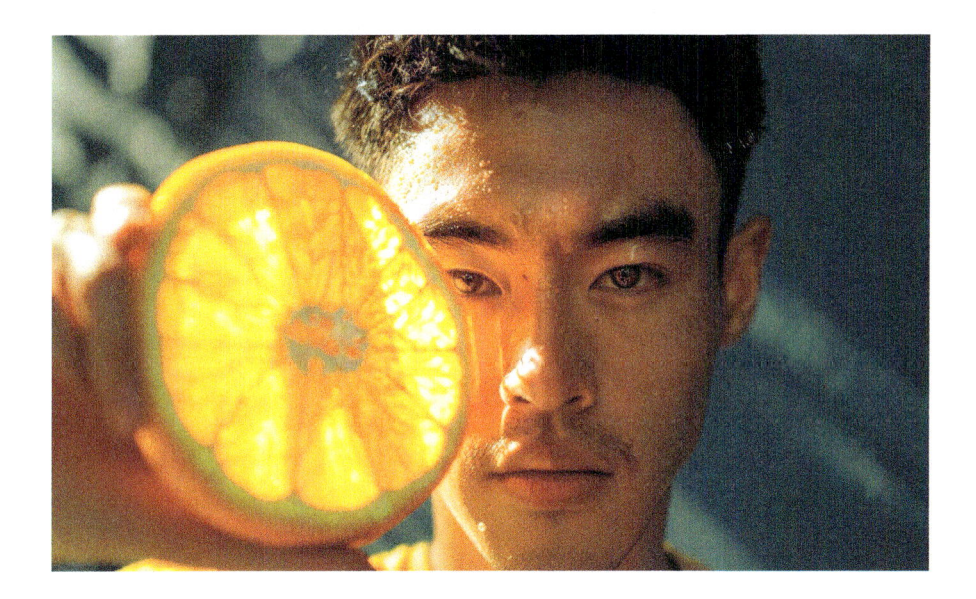

Vitamin C is often the star of the show regarding immune support. It's a powerful antioxidant that helps protect your cells from damage and is essential in producing white blood cells, which are critical players in your immune defense. Foods rich in vitamin C, including oranges, strawberries, bell peppers, and broccoli, are easy to find.

Including these foods in your diet isn't just about warding off the common cold; it's about ensuring your immune cells are healthy and ready to respond to threats.

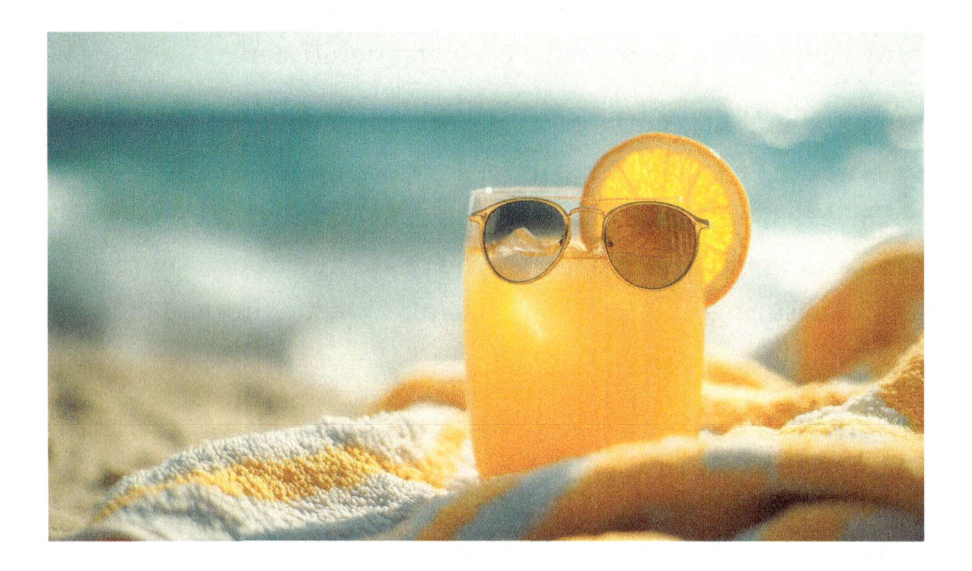

Then there's vitamin D, sometimes called the "sunshine vitamin" because your body produces it when exposed to sunlight. However, many of us don't get enough sun exposure, especially in the winter, making it essential to get vitamin D from our diet or supplements. Why is it crucial? Vitamin D is known for its role in bone health but is vital for immune function. It helps regulate the immune system and enhances the pathogen-fighting effects of monocytes and macrophages—white blood cells are essential to your immune defense. Fatty fish like salmon and mackerel, as well as fortified foods like milk and cereal, are good sources of vitamin D.

Zinc is another critical nutrient; it helps keep your immune system strong, aids in wound healing, and supports average growth. A zinc deficiency can significantly affect your immune system's ability to function correctly, leading to an increased risk of infection and disease. Zinc-rich foods include lean meats, poultry, seafood, milk, whole grain products, beans, seeds, and nuts. Integrating these into your diet helps ensure your immune system has the zinc to work effectively.

Selenium might not get as much attention, but it's equally important. This nutrient has powerful antioxidant properties that help lower oxidative stress in your body, reducing inflammation and enhancing immunity. Foods rich in selenium include garlic, broccoli, sardines, and tuna. These foods reduce inflammation and improve your daily requirement of selenium, making it easy to get this powerful nutrient into your diet.

ENHANCING GUT HEALTH AND IMMUNITY | 73

Now, let's talk about antioxidants. These substances protect your cells against free radicals, which are molecules that can cause harm and inflammation in the body. Berries are an excellent source of antioxidants; they boost your immune system, prevent tissue damage, and reduce the risk of chronic diseases. Nuts and green leafy vegetables like spinach and kale contain antioxidants and other nutrients that support immune health.

In addition to these nutrient-rich foods, herbs like echinacea, ginger, and turmeric can support your immune health. Echinacea is popular for its potential to pretense, while ginger has anti-inflammatory and intuitive properties, helping to reduce inflammation and enhance the immune response. Conversely, turmeric contains curcumin, a compound with potent anti-inflammatory properties that helps boost immune cell activity. Including these herbs in your cooking adds flavor and provides health benefits that bolster your body's defenses.

Building a meal plan incorporating these immune-boosting foods can be fun and beneficial. Start by thinking about meals that naturally include these elements.

A smoothie made with berries, orange juice, and a banana offers a potent dose of vitamin C and antioxidants for breakfast. Lunch could be a spinach salad with slices of turkey or salmon sprinkled with seeds for a zinc boost. For dinner, stir-fried broccoli and bell peppers with garlic and ginger chicken can make a delicious and nutrient-packed meal. Each meal is an opportunity to feed your immune system what it needs to protect you.

By understanding and utilizing these nutrients and foods, you're not just eating; you're fortifying your body's defenses and supporting them in keeping you healthy. This approach to diet takes the adage "you are what you eat" to a new level, showing that with the proper nutrients, you're building a stronger, more resilient you.

COMBATING COMMON DIGESTIVE ISSUES WITH DIET

When it comes to digestive health, several common issues can disrupt your day-to-day life, leaving you uncomfortable or even in pain. Conditions like irritable bowel syndrome (IBS), constipation, and acid reflux each come with their own set of challenges. IBS, for instance, often includes symptoms such as cramping, abdominal pain, bloating, gas, and either diarrhea or constipation. It's a rollercoaster and can be triggered by various factors, including diet and stress. Constipation, another common issue, involves having fewer than three bowel movements a week, often resulting in hard, dry stools that are difficult to pass. It's uncomfortable and can lead to significant bloating and discomfort. Acid reflux, or GERD, involves stomach acid flowing uncomfortably from your throat to your stomach, causing pain and a sour taste.

Adjusting your diet can be a powerful tool for managing these conditions. For those dealing with IBS, identifying and avoiding trigger foods is critical. Common triggers include high-gas foods like carbonated beverages and certain vegetables (broccoli, cauliflower), and large meals can also exacerbate symptoms. Instead, try incorporating low-FODMAP foods, as these are known to be easier on your digestive system. Increasing your fiber intake is beneficial for constipation as it helps keep things moving in your digestive tract. Foods rich in fiber, like fruits, vegetables, beans, and whole grains, can make a significant difference. Pair these with plenty of water to help soften stools and promote a healthy flow. Acid reflux sufferers will find relief by avoiding spicy and high-fat foods, which tend to increase stomach acid production. Instead, opt for lean meats, whole grains, and alkaline foods like bananas and melons that can help counteract stomach acid.

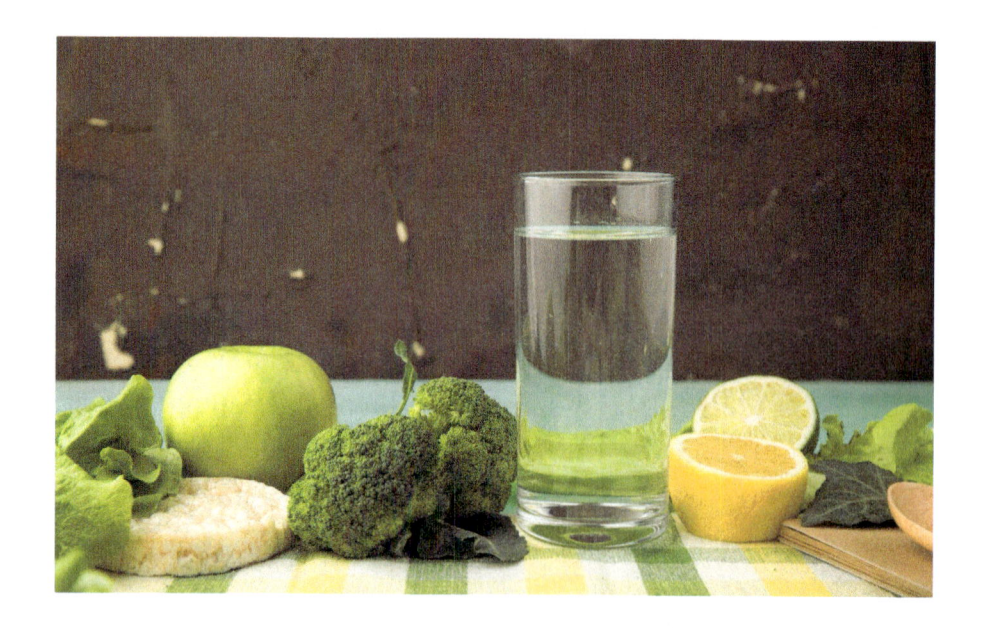

Hydration plays a crucial role in digestive health across the board. Water helps dissolve fats and soluble fiber, allowing these substances to pass through your intestines easily. For those dealing with constipation, proper hydration ensures that the fiber you consume can do its job effectively, helping to keep bowel movements regular. In the case of acid reflux, drinking water can help dilute and clear stomach acid from your esophagus, relieving symptoms. Aim for about 8–10 glasses of water daily, but remember that you might need more if you're active or live in a hot climate.

Sometimes, dietary adjustments and hydration might not be enough, and that's okay. It's important to recognize when professional help is needed. If you experience severe or persistent symptoms such as weight loss, blood in your stool, or unbearable abdominal pain, it's time to visit a healthcare provider. These could be signs of a more serious underlying condition that requires medical intervention. A healthcare provider can offer a diagnosis and specialized treatment options that can provide relief and help you manage your condition effectively. Remember, taking care of your digestive health is about easing current discomfort and preventing more serious health issues down the road. Keeping an eye on your body's signals and responding appropriately can help you maintain digestive health and overall well-being.

THE IMPACT OF STRESS ON GUT HEALTH AND IMMUNITY

Stress isn't just something you feel when you're rushing to meet a deadline or caught in traffic; it's also something that can profoundly affect your gut, creating a ripple effect on your overall health. When you're stressed, your body goes into 'fight or flight' mode, which can cause a slowdown in digestive processes as the body diverts energy to more critical functions. This change can affect gut motility—the movement of food through your digestive system—which can lead to issues like bloating, discomfort, and changes in bowel habits. Stress can also increase the permeability of your intestinal lining (often referred to as "leaky gut"), allowing bacteria and toxins to pass into the bloodstream, which can exacerbate inflammation and lead to further health complications like peptic ulcers and exacerbate conditions like irritable bowel syndrome (IBS).

Combating these effects can start with mindful eating, a practice that involves paying full attention to the experience of eating and drinking inside and outside the body. Mindful eating teaches you to notice how different foods affect your feelings and sensations in your body. It helps you recognize your body's hunger and fullness signals more clearly, which can prevent overeating and undue stress on your digestive system. Eating slowly and without distraction gives your body time to process what you're eating, which can help regulate your digestive processes and improve gut health.

Incorporating certain foods into your diet can also help mitigate the effects of stress on your body. Complex carbohydrates, for instance, aid in producing serotonin, a neurotransmitter that helps regulate mood, appetite, and digestion. Foods like oatmeal, whole grain bread, and brown rice are comforting and boost serotonin levels, helping to stabilize mood and reduce stress. Additionally, the fiber in these foods can promote a healthy gut microbiome, which is crucial for overall health.

However, managing stress isn't just about changing what you eat; it's also about incorporating regular stress-reduction practices into your life. Techniques like yoga, meditation, and regular physical activity can be incredibly effective.

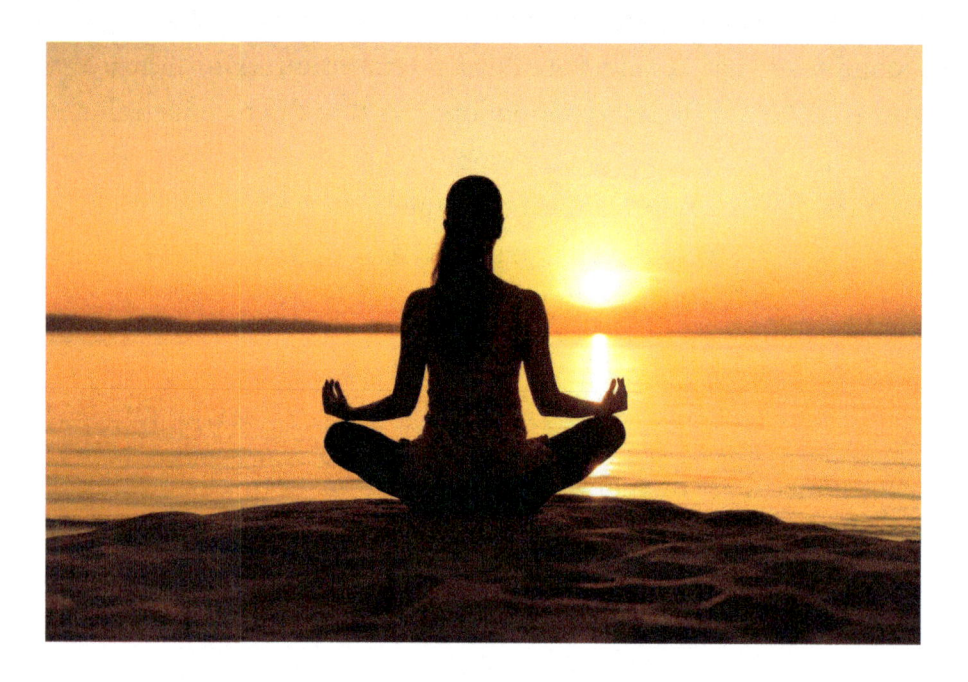

Yoga combines physical postures, breathing exercises, and meditation to enhance physical and mental health, which can help reduce stress and its adverse impacts on gut health. Meditation, even for a few minutes a day, can help reduce stress and anxiety by bringing about relaxation and calm. Regular physical activity, be it a brisk walk, a run, or a dance class, helps release endorphins, the body's natural painkillers, and mood elevators, which can improve gut motility and overall digestive health.

Understanding how stress affects your gut and integrating stress-reducing foods and practices into your daily routine can help protect your digestive system from the harmful effects of stress and improve your overall well-being. Remember, taking care of your gut is not just about what you eat; it's also about managing stress, practicing mindfulness, and staying active, all of which are crucial in maintaining a healthy, happy gut.

LIFESTYLE CHANGES TO SUPPORT DIGESTIVE HEALTH

Embracing a few lifestyle tweaks can significantly enhance your digestive health, turning your gut into a well-oiled machine and supporting overall wellness. Let's explore how regular physical activity, quality sleep, avoiding harmful habits, and a consistent daily routine can foster a healthier digestive system.

Regular exercise is a fantastic way to keep your digestive system running smoothly. You might not realize it, but staying active goes beyond just keeping you fit—it's also essential for promoting gut motility, which is food movement through your digestive tract. When you exercise, your body's natural rhythm enhances this movement, helping to prevent issues like constipation and bloating. It's like giving your internal plumbing a good workout, ensuring everything flows as it should. Furthermore, regular physical activity increases the diversity of beneficial bacteria in your gut, which is crucial for digestion, your immune system, and mental health. Incorporating activities like walking, cycling, or yoga into your daily routine can significantly affect how your gut functions, making you feel lighter and more vibrant.

Now, let's talk about the impact of sleep on your digestive health. Sleep, including your digestive system, is the body's time to repair and rejuvenate. A lack of quality sleep can increase the stress hormone cortisol, which may disrupt your gut flora and create a cascade of digestive issues, including increased sensitivity and inflammation. Aim for 7–9 hours of sleep daily to support your digestive health. Creating a bedtime routine can help signal your body that it's time to wind down. Activities like reading, taking a warm bath, or practicing relaxation exercises might be included. Also, try to keep your bedtime and wake-up times consistent, even on weekends, to regulate your body's internal clock, which can help improve your sleep quality and, consequently, your digestion.

Avoiding harmful habits such as smoking, excessive alcohol consumption, and too much caffeine is crucial for maintaining a healthy gut. These substances can irritate your gastrointestinal lining, leading to inflammation and other digestive issues. To protect your gut health, consider gradually reducing these habits. For instance, if you're used to having several cups of coffee daily, try replacing some of those with herbal teas or water. Not only will this reduce your caffeine intake, but staying well-hydrated is vital to keeping things moving smoothly in your digestive tract.

Lastly, establishing a routine that supports regular meal times can significantly benefit your digestive health. Eating meals at similar times daily can help regulate your body's digestive system. Think of it as setting a schedule that your gut can get used to. Regular meal times can prevent a range of issues, from indigestion to bloating, as they allow your digestive system to prepare for and optimize the process of digestion and nutrient absorption. Plus, when your body knows when to expect food, it can manage energy more effectively throughout the day, keeping you more balanced and energized.

Integrating these lifestyle changes—increasing physical activity, improving sleep quality, avoiding detrimental habits, and establishing a consistent daily routine—creates an environment that supports optimum digestive function. These habits help you cultivate a resilient digestive system that functions efficiently and supports your overall health and well-being.

As we close this chapter on enhancing gut health and immunity, remember that your digestive health is deeply intertwined with your overall lifestyle choices. Maintaining a healthy digestive system relies on various aspects, including your activities, the rest you take, and the routines you establish. As we move forward, we'll explore how to overcome challenges and stay motivated by equipping you to maintain your health through informed, practical choices. Let's build on this foundation, enhance your knowledge, and empower you to take control of your health in the most fulfilling ways.

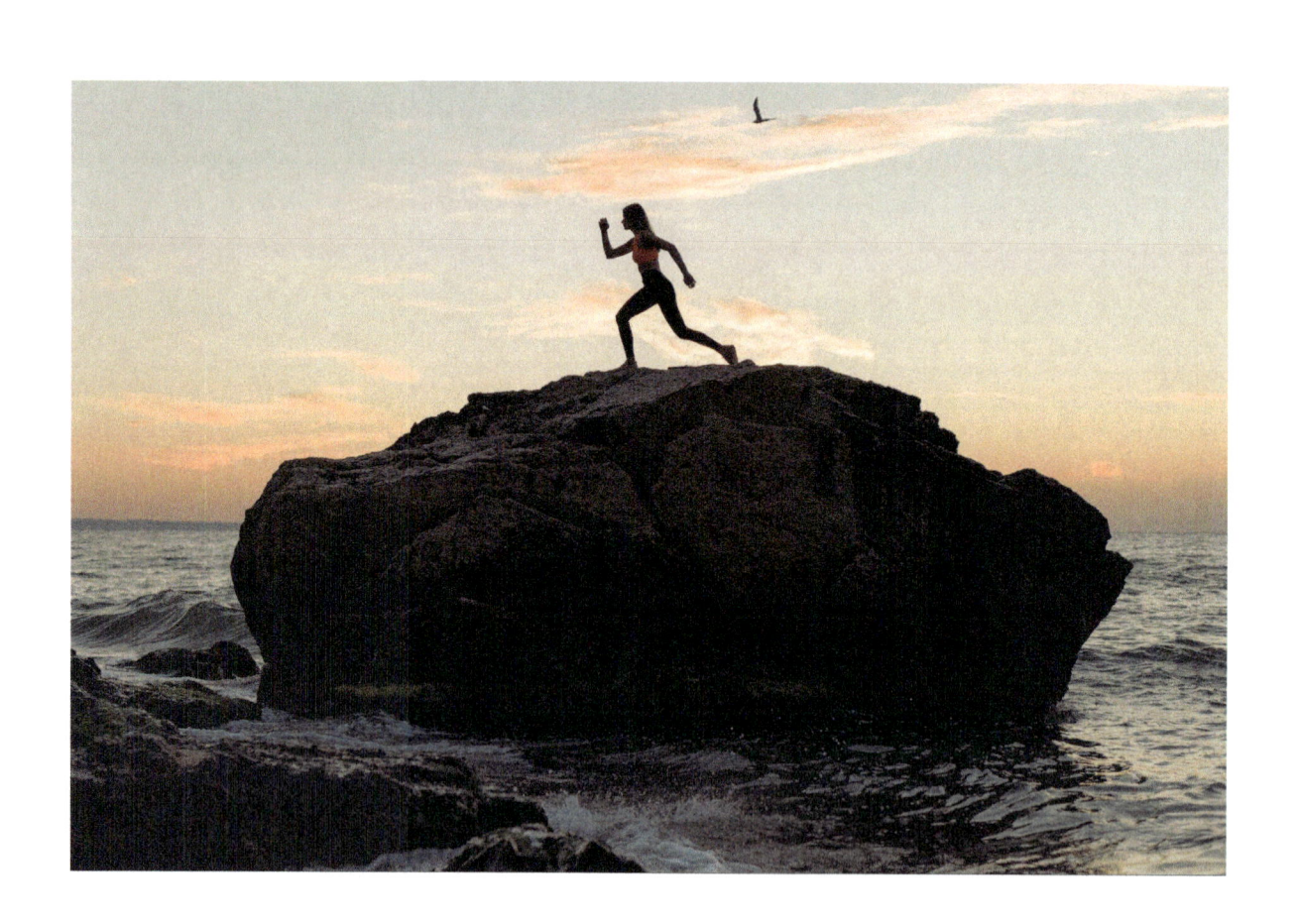

6

OVERCOMING CHALLENGES AND STAYING MOTIVATED

Ah, the social scene! It's where food and fun intersect, but if you're on an anti-inflammatory diet, navigating social gatherings, family dinners, and everything in between can sometimes feel like you're a sailboat trying to steer through stormy weather. Don't worry, though! With a few intelligent strategies up your sleeve, you can easily sail through these social waters, keeping your diet on track without missing out on the fun.

DEALING WITH SOCIAL AND FAMILY DINING CHALLENGES

Navigating Social Events

Imagine being invited to a big bash with a tempting spread. One effective strategy is to eat a healthy meal before heading out. This way, you're not arriving with an empty stomach, which could make it hard to resist less healthy options. Think of it as putting on your dietary armor. Another great tactic is sharing a dish that fits your anti-inflammatory diet.

Not only does this ensure there's something you can enjoy, but it also introduces your friends to the delicious possibilities of your diet. Who knows? Your quinoa salad or roasted veggies might just steal the show!

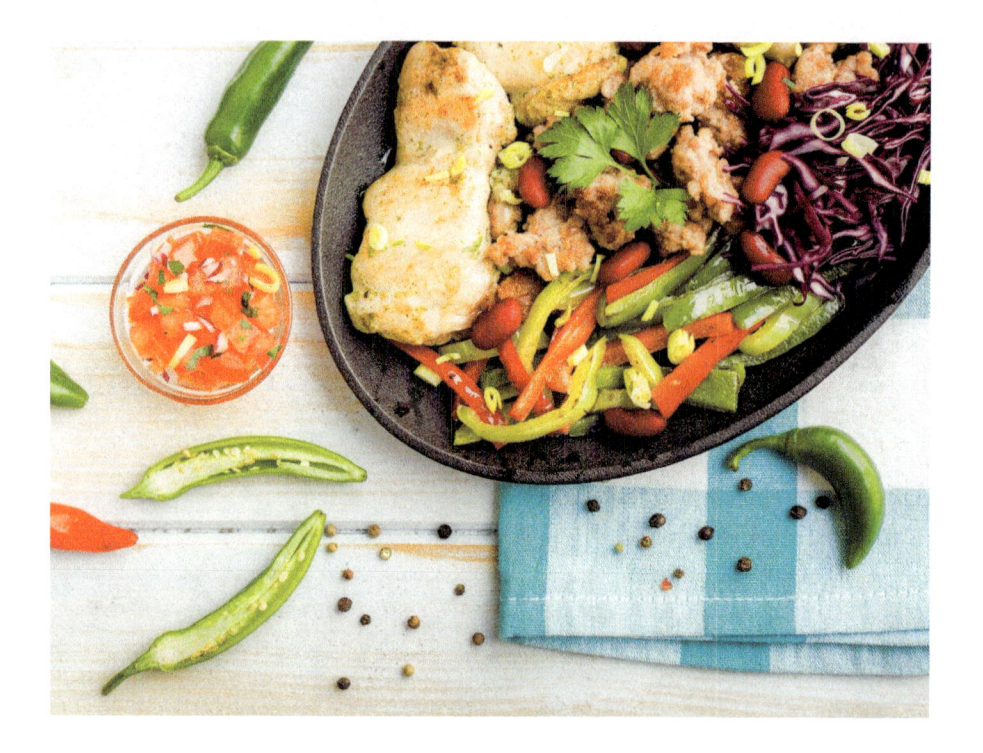

Communicating Dietary Needs

Being open about your dietary needs with hosts or when you're a guest at someone's home is also essential. Most people will appreciate your honesty and might even go the extra mile to accommodate your needs. The key here is clarity and respect—explain your dietary restrictions with a smile and express your appreciation for their effort. It's not about demanding special treatment but about making your needs known in a way that also considers your host's feelings.

Inclusive Meal Planning

Regarding family meals, inclusivity is the name of the game. You want to prepare dishes everyone can enjoy, regardless of whether they follow an anti-inflammatory diet. Start with a base dish everyone loves and tweak it to fit your dietary needs. For example, if your family loves spaghetti, you might use whole wheat or lentil pasta and whip up a sauce bursting with anti-inflammatory herbs like basil and oregano. Let family members customize their plates with add-ons like cheese or chili flakes. This way, everyone feels part of the meal without the need to prepare completely separate dishes.

Handling Peer Pressure

Finally, let's talk about handling peer pressure. It can be challenging when friends or colleagues urge you to "try a bite" or question your dietary choices. Stand your ground with a polite but firm response. You might say, "I've found that eating this way improves how I feel daily, but I appreciate your offer!" Remember, staying true to your diet and health goals are something to be proud of, not shy away from. It's about your well-being—something worth sticking to, even under a little social pressure.

Navigating the social aspects of dieting is as much about communication and planning as it is about the food itself. By preparing ahead, engaging openly and honestly with others about your needs, and finding inclusive ways to enjoy meals together, you transform potential dietary challenges into opportunities for sharing and connection. Making it easier and more enjoyable to stick to your anti-inflammatory diet involves integrating healthy habits into all aspects of your social life.

FINDING QUICK FIXES FOR BUSY DAYS

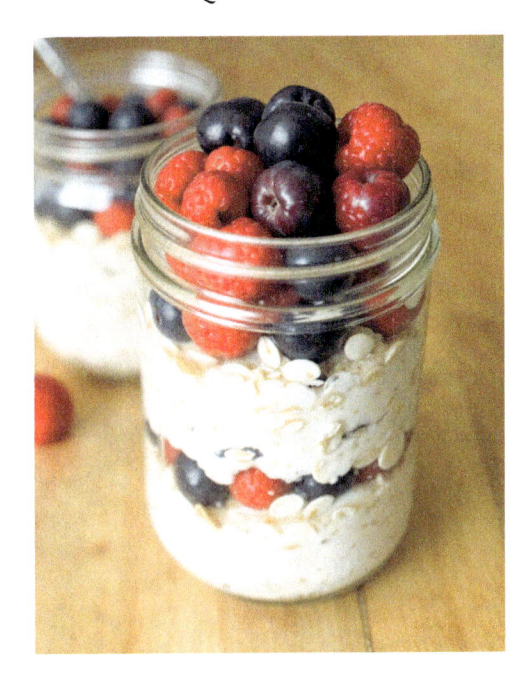

Life's pace just keeps quickening, doesn't it? Sometimes, even preparing a simple meal feels like a mountain of a task. Who said quick can't be healthy? Let's dive into some nifty tricks and tips that ensure you stick to your anti-inflammatory diet, no matter how packed your schedule gets.

First off, let's talk about preprepared meal ideas. Imagine having a fridge full of ready-to-go meals that align with your health goals. It's doable and a game-changer for your busy days. Think about meals that are easy to prepare and store well. Overnight oats can be a fantastic breakfast option. Just mix rolled oats with almond milk, chia seeds, and some berries, and let it sit in the fridge overnight. Voila, a creamy, nutritious breakfast awaits you in the morning!

For lunch, how about mason jar salads? Layer some leafy greens, chopped veggies, a good protein source like grilled chicken or chickpeas, and a light dressing. When you're ready to eat, just shake it up. These meals aren't just quick; they ensure you get a good dose of anti-inflammatory foods with minimal effort.

Navigating fast-food menus for healthier options can also be tricky, but many popular fast-food joints now offer better choices that fit into an anti-inflammatory diet. Look for grilled items over fried, salads with lots of veggies and lean proteins, and sides like apple slices or yogurt. Always opt for water or unsweetened iced tea instead of soda. These choices can help you maintain your diet when you're in a pinch for time and need to grab something on the go.

Now, let's talk about the tools of the trade. Efficient kitchen gadgets are like your best friends in the kitchen. A good blender can do wonders.

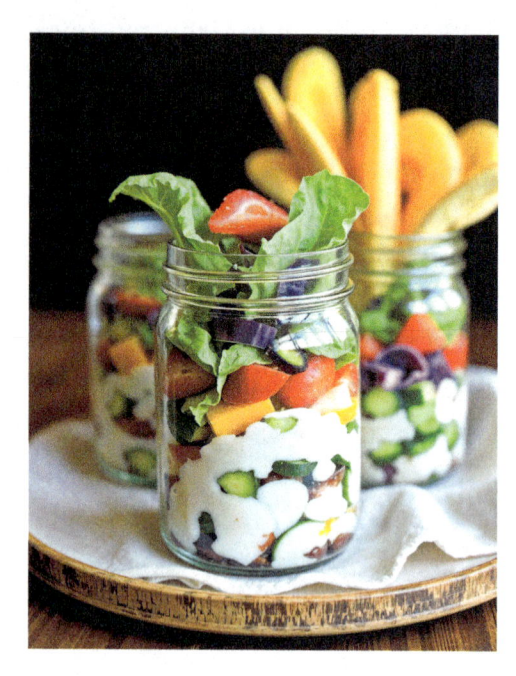

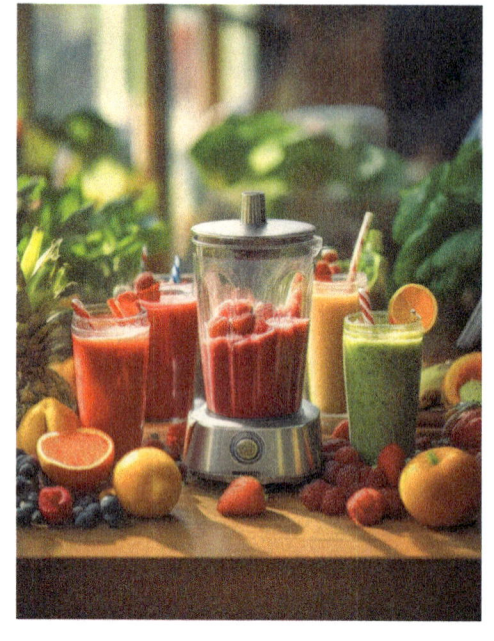

Smoothies are a quick, nutritious option that can serve as a meal or a filling snack, and with the right blender, they're a breeze to make. Throw in some spinach, a small banana, a handful of berries, some flaxseed, and your choice of milk or juice, and you've got a potent anti-inflammatory drink in minutes. Another superhero gadget is the pressure cooker. It dramatically reduces cooking time and can be used for various dishes. Think stews, soups, and steamed vegetables, all rich in nutrients and prepared in less than half the time it would typically take.

Lastly, efficient time management can revolutionize your meal prep process. It might sound mundane, but planning your weekly meals can save time and stress. Spend a little time each week to map out your meals.

Check what ingredients you already have and what you need to buy. It not only saves time while grocery shopping but also minimizes waste. Organizing your cooking space can also streamline the cooking process. Keep your most-used tools and ingredients within easy reach, and maintain a clear, clutter-free countertop. This setup reduces preparation time and makes the cooking process more enjoyable.

Incorporating these strategies into your routine can help you maintain your anti-inflammatory diet without feeling like a chore, even on your busiest days. With some planning and tools, you can create quick, healthy meals that support your health and fit into your fast-paced life. Remember, every small step in consciously preparing and choosing meals significantly contributes to your wellness journey.

HANDLING CRAVINGS AND COMFORT FOOD ALTERNATIVES

Cravings can be quite the problem, right? They hit you out of nowhere, making you yearn for something sweet, salty, or downright decadent—even when you're not hungry. Understanding the roots of these cravings is key to managing them effectively. Often, cravings are not just about hunger; they're a complex interplay of psychological and physiological factors. Sometimes, they reflect our emotional states—boredom, stress, sadness, or even joy can trigger cravings for foods we associate with comfort or reward. Physiologically, cravings can also arise from fluctuations in blood sugar levels or hormonal changes. For instance, dips in serotonin levels, a hormone that boosts mood, can make you crave carbohydrates because they help produce serotonin.

Distinguishing between true hunger and emotional eating is crucial. If you've eaten a balanced meal not too long ago and still find yourself stalking the kitchen, it's likely a craving rather than hunger. A good strategy here is to pause and ask yourself what you feel. Is it hunger, or is it boredom or stress? This pause can help you make a conscious decision rather than dive headfirst into a bag of chips.

Healthy swaps can be a lifesaver when cravings strike—craving something crunchy and salty like chips? Baked sweet potato fries might hit the spot without derailing your anti-inflammatory diet. They're tasty and satisfying and offer a good dose of nutrients. Sweet cravings can be more challenging, especially if you've got a serious sweet tooth. Instead of reaching for ice cream, how about blending some frozen bananas with vanilla for a creamy, dreamy treat? Top it with a sprinkle of cinnamon or a few dark chocolate chips, and you've got yourself a dessert that's both satisfying and aligned with your health goals.

Creating satisfying and flavorful meals is another effective strategy to combat cravings. It's not just about filling your belly but satisfying your taste buds, too. Start with a good protein source, like grilled chicken or tofu, add a complex carbohydrate like quinoa or sweet potatoes, and pile on the veggies. Dress it up with spices and herbs—turmeric, ginger, basil, or mint can add a punch of flavor and anti-inflammatory benefits. When your meals are balanced and tasty, you're less likely to feel deprived and more likely to feel content, which naturally reduces cravings.

Mindful eating is a powerful practice that helps manage cravings. It involves entirely focusing on the eating experience—savoring each bite, recognizing the flavors, and listening to your body's hunger and fullness cues. This practice enhances mealtime satisfaction and helps you realize when you eat out of emotion rather than hunger. Next time you sit down to a meal, try this: Take a small bite, put your fork down, and taste your food. Notice the texture, the flavors, and how it makes you feel. Slowing down your eating pace can increase enjoyment and help you feel more satisfied with smaller portions.

You can navigate cravings without falling off the anti-inflammatory wagon by understanding the roots of your cravings, employing smart food swaps, crafting satisfying meals, and practicing mindful eating. These strategies are not just about resisting temptation; they're about creating a new, healthier relationship with food where you're in control and each meal brings you joy and health.

CELEBRATING SUCCESS: REWARDING YOUR DIETARY ACHIEVEMENTS

When you've committed to an anti-inflammatory diet, every step you take is a victory worth celebrating. Think of your diet as a series of milestones, not just a finish line. Setting realistic goals along the way and giving yourself a pat on the back when you meet them isn't just rewarding; it's crucial for maintaining motivation. Let's say you've decided to integrate more leafy greens into your meals, and after a week, you've managed to do just that at every dinner. That's a fantastic achievement! Celebrate these small victories because they add to significant health benefits over time. It might help to write down these goals and tick them off as you achieve them, which can be incredibly satisfying and encouraging.

Now, about those celebrations—while it might be tempting to treat yourself to a sugary dessert or a fancy dinner, why not think outside the box of edible rewards? Nonfood rewards can be equally, if not more, gratifying. Perhaps treat yourself to a spa day after a month of sticking to your anti-inflammatory meal plans, or buy new workout gear to inspire your next phase of healthy living. Even planning a day trip to a nearby city or nature reserve can be a fantastic way to reward yourself. These experiences celebrate your success and enhance your overall well-being, aligning perfectly with your healthier, more balanced life goals.

Reflecting on your progress regularly is another essential element in this journey. It's easy to forget how far you've come, especially when you need to see the immediate benefits. Take a moment each week to reflect on what you've accomplished, how you feel physically and mentally, and any improvements in symptoms you've noticed. Maybe you've had less joint pain, or you find yourself with more energy in the mornings. Documenting these changes, perhaps in a journal or a digital diary, can provide a motivational boost. Reading back through your progress can be incredibly uplifting on days when you need a reminder of why you started this path in the first place.

Sharing your success stories plays a dual role. Not only does it reinforce your commitment by vocalizing your achievements, but it can also inspire others to consider their health and explore an anti-inflammatory diet. Whether through social media, a blog, or just chatting with friends, sharing your journey can lead to a supportive community that cheers each other on. Hearing how others have benefited from similar changes can reinforce the positive impacts of your efforts, making the diet feel less like a personal challenge and more like a shared, communal lifestyle shift.

As you continue to set and reach your dietary milestones, remember that each step forward is part of a larger picture of health and happiness. By celebrating these achievements, reflecting on your progress, and sharing your journey, you maintain the motivation to continue and the joy and satisfaction of living well.

BUILDING A SUPPORT NETWORK: ONLINE AND OFFLINE

Embarking on an anti-inflammatory diet can sometimes feel like venturing into uncharted waters. Having a solid support network can make these waters much smoother to navigate. It's not just about having people around who understand what you're going through; it's also about creating a community that inspires and motivates you, providing a safety net on those days when your motivation might wane. Whether online or offline, the proper support can make all the difference in maintaining your dietary changes and enjoying the journey.

The internet is bustling with forums, social media groups, and blogs dedicated to anti-inflammatory lifestyles, starting with the digital world. These platforms can be invaluable resources for connecting with others committed to reducing inflammation through diet. Imagine having a rough day; maybe you slipped up at a social event or felt overwhelmed by dietary choices. A quick post in one of these groups can offer comfort, practical advice, and encouragement to get back on track. Websites like Reddit and Facebook host numerous groups where members share recipe success stories and even organize meet-ups. If you're looking for recipe inspiration or need advice on handling a particular challenge, these communities can be just a click away. Plus, the anonymity and accessibility of online forums often make it easier to share and ask questions without feeling self-conscious.

On the flip side, local support groups offer a more personal touch. These are people you can meet regularly, share meals with, and get to know on a deeper level. To find such groups, check community boards at local health food stores, libraries, or community centers. Many areas have wellness groups focused on various aspects of health, including diet and inflammation. Joining a group can provide you with emotional and moral support and a sense of accountability, which can be incredibly motivating. Additionally, many cities have wellness events or health fairs focusing on nutrition and healthy living. Attending these events can help you connect with like-minded individuals and find professional nutritionists or dietitians specializing in anti-inflammatory diets.

Involving your friends and family in your dietary journey can also be crucial to success. Start by inviting them to try out new recipes with you, perhaps during a weekly dinner date. Cooking together can be fun and engaging to introduce your loved ones to your lifestyle changes. It's also an excellent opportunity to explain the reasons behind your dietary choices, which can help them better understand and support your goals. If they're curious, share articles or books that have been helpful to you. Sometimes, seeing the science behind your dietary choices can turn skepticism into support.

Lastly, I always appreciate the value of professional support. A dietitian or a nutritionist, especially one specializing in anti-inflammatory diets, can offer guidance tailored to your needs. They can help refine your diet, suggest supplements, and monitor your progress, providing adjustments along the way. If you have underlying health issues or find that navigating the diet on your own is challenging, this professional guidance can be crucial. Finding the right professional might seem daunting, but you can start by seeking referrals from your healthcare provider or local wellness centers. A good professional will provide support and empower you with the knowledge to make informed dietary choices.

Building a robust support network is essential for anyone embarking on a diet that requires significant lifestyle changes. Whether it's sharing a recipe, getting a pep talk when you're feeling down, or receiving professional advice, the proper support can make your dietary journey smoother and more enjoyable. With each interaction, whether online or in person, you gain support and build lifelong friendships and connections beyond food.

STAYING INSPIRED: CONTINUOUSLY REFRESHING YOUR MEAL PLANS

Keeping your meal plan vibrant and enticing is crucial when adhering to an anti-inflammatory diet. It's easy to follow a routine of repeating the same meals, but let's spice things up a bit! Exploring new recipes and cuisines can turn what might start to feel like a dietary routine into an exciting culinary adventure. Picture this: You could travel the globe from your kitchen each week! Try incorporating dishes from different cultures that align with anti-inflammatory guidelines—perhaps a Thai curry packed with anti-inflammatory ginger and turmeric or a Moroccan stew with plenty of anti-inflammatory spices like cinnamon and cumin. These dishes don't just ignite your taste buds; they bring new nutrients and benefits, keeping your diet balanced and exciting.

Diving into the world of seasonal eating can also rejuvenate your meal plan. Each season offers a bounty of fresh produce, which can inspire new dishes and flavors. Salads with fresh berries, cucumbers, and tomatoes can be your go-to meals in summer, light yet satisfying. When autumn rolls around, it's time for hearty soups and stews with squash and kale. Winter could introduce you to the warming comfort of roasted root vegetables, while spring brings the crisp freshness of asparagus and peas. Seasonal eating not only injects variety into your diet but also ensures you're getting produce at its peak nutritional value, not to mention it's often more environmentally friendly and economical to buy foods that are in season.

Now, let's talk about keeping your anti-inflammatory knowledge fresh. Immersing yourself in educational resources like books, documentaries, and cooking shows focused on anti-inflammatory eating can inspire and motivate you. For instance, watching a cooking show focusing on healthy cuisine can introduce you to new cooking techniques and ingredient combinations you might not have considered before. Attending workshops or virtual webinars about nutrition and health can deepen your understanding and commitment to your dietary choices, keeping you engaged and informed.

Lastly, why not make meal planning a fun challenge? Engage with friends or online community members in recipe challenges, where you might pick an ingredient for the week that everyone creates a dish around. Sharing results online can be fun, as it can be fun to see how different people interpret the same ingredient, providing you with new ideas and a sense of community. Making the dietary process enjoyable integrates it into your social activities, enriching your experience and broadening your culinary horizons.

By continuously exploring new recipes, embracing the rhythm of seasonal eating, educating yourself with engaging resources, and turning meal preparation into a shared challenge, you ensure that your anti-inflammatory diet remains a dynamic and integral part of your life. This approach keeps your meals exciting and helps maintain your commitment to a healthy lifestyle, making your dietary routine not just about health but also pleasure and discovery.

As we wrap up this chapter on overcoming challenges and staying motivated, remember that the key to sustaining any long-term dietary change is to keep things fresh, engaging, and enjoyable. Whether exploring new recipes, incorporating seasonal foods, educating yourself, or turning meal prep into a fun challenge, each strategy plays a vital role in keeping you motivated and committed to your anti-inflammatory diet. By embracing these approaches, you ensure that your journey is healthy but also rich and fulfilling. Now, let's move forward and continue to build on the foundation we've set, exploring further how to sustain and adapt these practices in everyday life in our upcoming chapter.

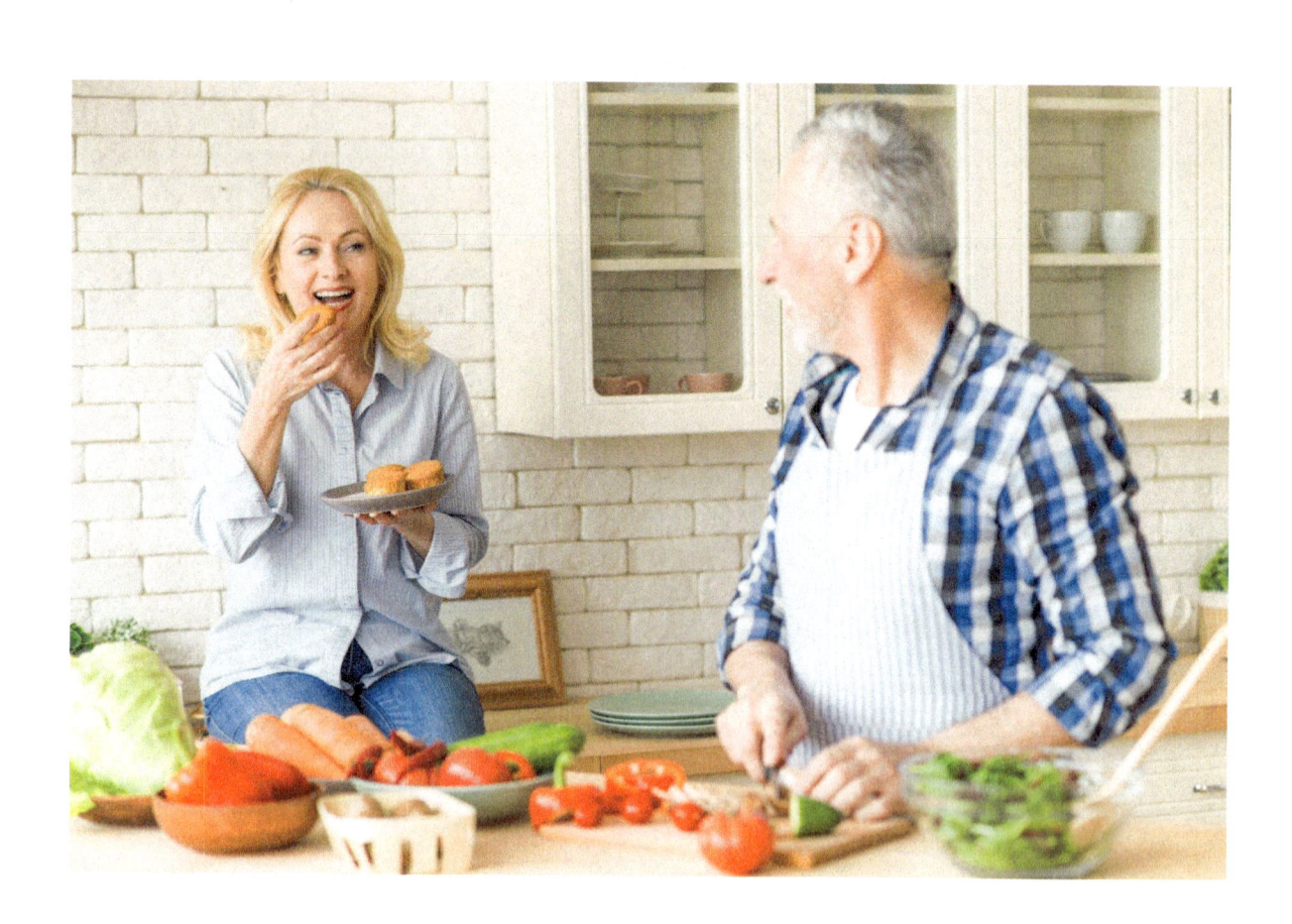

7

SUSTAINING AN ANTI-INFLAMMATORY LIFESTYLE LONG-TERM

Stepping into a healthier lifestyle isn't just about adjusting what's on your plate; it's about moving your body, too! Merging a thoughtful, anti-inflammatory diet with regular physical activity isn't just a boon for your waistline; it's a powerhouse combo for your overall health. Here, we'll dive into how these elements work better together, like a well-oiled machine, enhancing everything from your heart health to your mood and ensuring you're living longer and better.

INTEGRATING PHYSICAL ACTIVITY FOR COMPREHENSIVE BENEFITS

The Synergy Between Diet and Exercise

Imagine your body as a complex network of systems that work in harmony. When you fuel it with anti-inflammatory foods, you're reducing internal inflammation and setting the stage for optimal functioning. But when you add exercise to the mix, you amplify these benefits. Exercise itself acts as an anti-inflammatory agent. It may sound counterintuitive, given the minor wear and tear it brings about, but this physical stress is good. It encourages your body to build more robust, efficient systems and helps flush out inflammation through increased circulation and the production of supportive biochemicals. For instance, a brisk walk can boost the production of antioxidants, which help protect your cells from damage, while strength training enhances muscle function and metabolism. Together, a balanced diet and regular exercise can significantly improve cardiovascular health, stabilize blood sugar, elevate your mood, and boost energy levels, making each day brighter and more productive than the last.

Types of Beneficial Exercises

Not all forms of exercise are created equal, especially when fighting inflammation. Activities like yoga, swimming, and moderate aerobic exercises are particularly potent. With its gentle stretches and focus on breathing, yoga reduces physical inflammation and alleviates stress, a significant contributor to inflammation. Swimming is another excellent option, especially if you're looking for a low-impact exercise that soothes and strengthens the joints instead of straining them. Aerobic activities like walking, cycling, or light jogging help improve blood flow and reduce specific inflammatory markers, such as CRP (C-reactive protein). These activities are flexible and can be adjusted to fit any lifestyle or fitness level, making them ideal for anyone starting their physical activity journey or looking for variety.

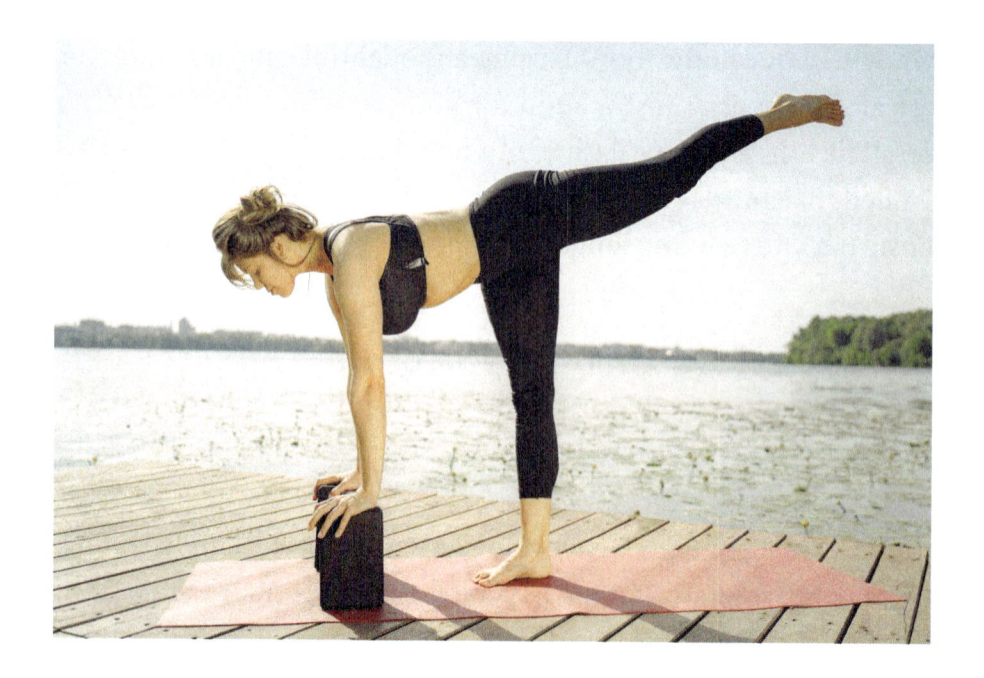

Setting a Routine

Consistency is the golden thread in the fabric of any successful health endeavor. It's not just about going hard at the gym or sticking strictly to salads but about setting a routine that blends seamlessly with your life. Start small—maybe a 10-minute walk after dinner or a morning yoga session—and gradually increase the duration and intensity as your body adapts. The key is to make it a habit, something as integral to your day as brushing your teeth. If you're struggling to find time, look at your schedule. Can you wake up 30 minutes earlier? Perhaps turn part of your lunch break into a brisk walk? Even short bursts of exercise, known as high-intensity interval training (HIIT), can be highly effective and easily fit into a busy schedule.

Overcoming Exercise Barriers

Let's face it: Starting and maintaining an exercise routine can be daunting, especially when faced with time constraints or a lack of motivation. If finding time is challenging, consider integrating physical activities into your daily routine. Instead of driving to the store, could you walk or cycle? You could do body-weight exercises like squats or sit-ups while watching TV. A lack of motivation can be more challenging, but setting clear, achievable goals can help. Whether improving your stamina, losing weight, or enhancing your overall health, having a clear target can make all the difference. And don't forget, exercising with friends or family can make the activity more enjoyable and keep you accountable. Sometimes, a little companionship is all you need to turn exercise from a chore into a highlight of your day.

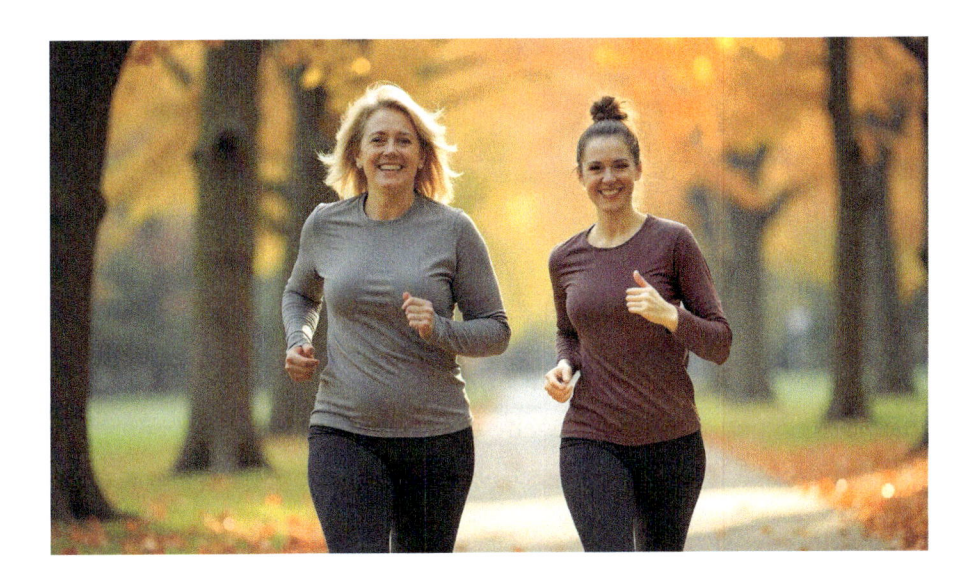

Integrating these physical activities into your routine and understanding how they complement your anti-inflammatory diet sets the stage for sustained health and vitality. It's not just about living longer; it's about enhancing the quality of your life and enabling you to enjoy each moment with more energy, less pain, and a clearer mind.

So, lace up your sneakers, unroll that yoga mat, or dive into the pool; your body (and mind) will thank you!

MINDFULNESS AND ITS ROLE IN ANTI-INFLAMMATORY EATING

Mindfulness might sound like a buzzword that's all the rage in wellness circles, but it's a simple practice with profound benefits, mainly when applied to eating. At its core, mindfulness is about being fully present and engaged with the current moment. Using this to eat means paying attention to your food, how it tastes and makes you feel, and the signals your body sends about hunger and satisfaction. It's about observing without judgment whether the food you choose is nurturing or depleting your body. This awareness can transform your relationship with food from mindless eating to a more intentional, health-supporting practice. Mindful eating encourages you to slow down, chew thoroughly, and truly savor each bite, leading to better digestion and greater enjoyment of your meals. It also helps you become acutely aware of your body's hunger and fullness cues, which can prevent overeating and make making choices that align with your anti-inflammatory goals easier.

The practice of eating without distractions is a critical component of mindful eating. In today's fast-paced world, eating while distracted is common—watching TV, scrolling through smartphones, or working through lunch. These distractions diminish the pleasure of eating and disconnect you from your body's natural cues. You can enhance your digestive processes by removing these distractions and focusing solely on your meal. Digestion begins in the brain, triggered by the sight and smell of food, which prepares your body to metabolize what you're about to consume. By paying attention to your meal, you're priming your body for optimal digestion and nutrient absorption and likely finding more satisfaction in smaller portions.

Extending mindfulness to selecting and preparing food also enriches the eating experience. When you shop and cook mindfully, you're more likely to make good choices for your body and the planet. Selecting locally grown produce supports local farmers and reduces your carbon footprint. Additionally, choosing organic options helps you avoid pesticides that contribute to inflammation. Taking the time to prepare your food thoughtfully can also be a meditative and enjoyable process. It allows you to connect with the journey of your food from source to table, deepening your appreciation for the nourishment it provides. Cooking becomes less of a chore and a creative, fulfilling practice that feeds your body and soul.

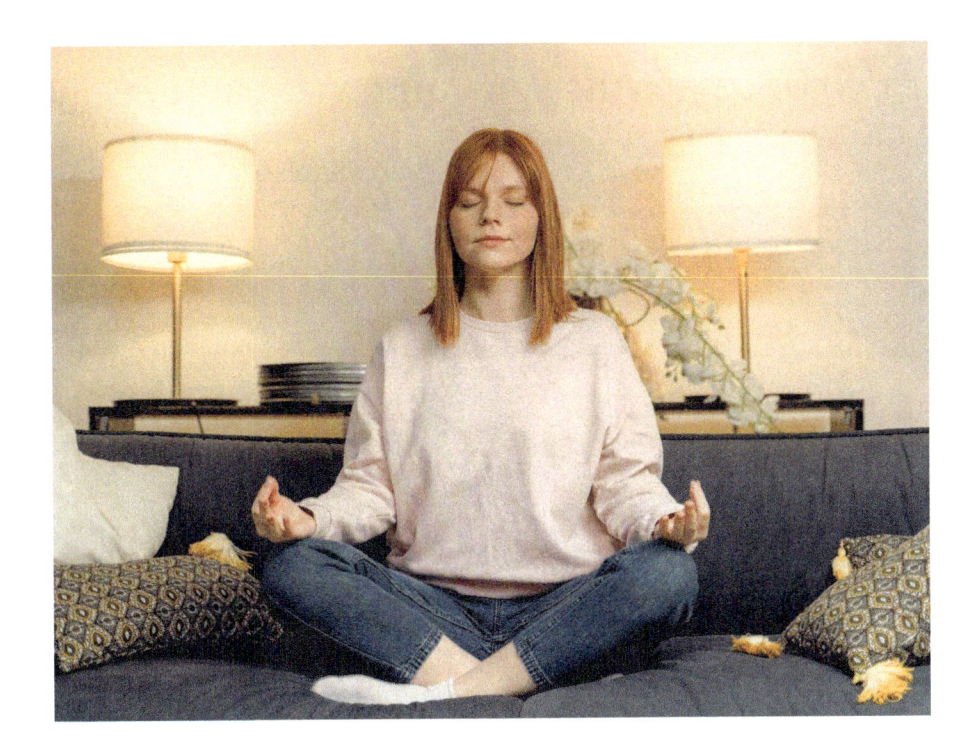

Mindfulness also offers a powerful tool for stress reduction, which is crucial since stress is a known trigger for inflammation. Integrating mindful practices like meditation and deep breathing into your daily routine can help you manage stress effectively. Meditation doesn't have to be daunting; it can be as simple as spending a few minutes each morning or evening sitting quietly, focusing on your breath, and releasing the thoughts that crowd your mind.

These practices help reduce stress and enhance your overall mindfulness, making it easier to maintain a calm, centered state throughout the day. This heightened sense of peace can make it easier to stick to your anti-inflammatory diet, as you're less likely to turn to comfort foods in response to stress.

By embracing mindfulness in eating, shopping, cooking, and managing stress, you create a supportive environment for your anti-inflammatory lifestyle. This approach doesn't just help you eat better; it enhances your entire way of being, leading to improved health, greater joy, and a deeper connection with the food that nourishes you. As you continue practicing mindfulness, it naturally extends into other areas of your life, offering a profound sense of presence and contentment beyond your meals.

SEASONAL EATING: ADJUSTING YOUR DIET WITH THE CALENDAR

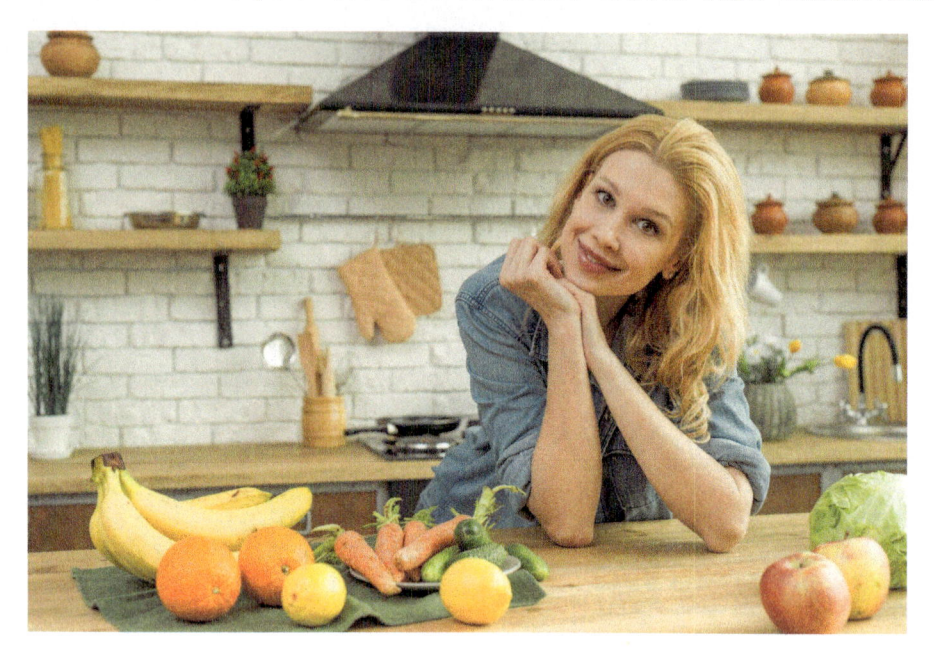

Eating with the seasons isn't just a charming old-school concept; it's a powerful way to enhance your health and tread more lightly on the planet. When you eat fruits and vegetables in their peak season, you get them at their nutritional best and their most flavorful. Seasonal produce often requires less human intervention, such as extensive use of pesticides and fertilizers, making it better for the environment. Additionally, buying local seasonal produce reduces the demand for shipping foods from far away, which lowers your carbon footprint. It's like giving the planet a little hug whenever you shop and dine. Plus, seasonal fruits and veggies tend to be more affordable when they're abundant. So, it's a win-win-win—better quality, lower cost, and environmentally friendly.

Now, you might wonder how to incorporate more seasonal foods into your diet. It's simpler than you might think! Start by doing a little research on what grows in your area during the seasons. Many websites and apps provide this information at a glance. Once you know what's likely to be in season, visiting local farmers' markets can be a delightful and eye-opening experience. Here, you can talk directly to growers to find out more about the produce they offer. These markets are often a treasure trove of local, seasonal produce, and most farmers are happy to share recipes or tips on preparing their products. Plus, the produce you find here is often fresher and richer in nutrients than in supermarkets, as it hasn't had to travel long distances.

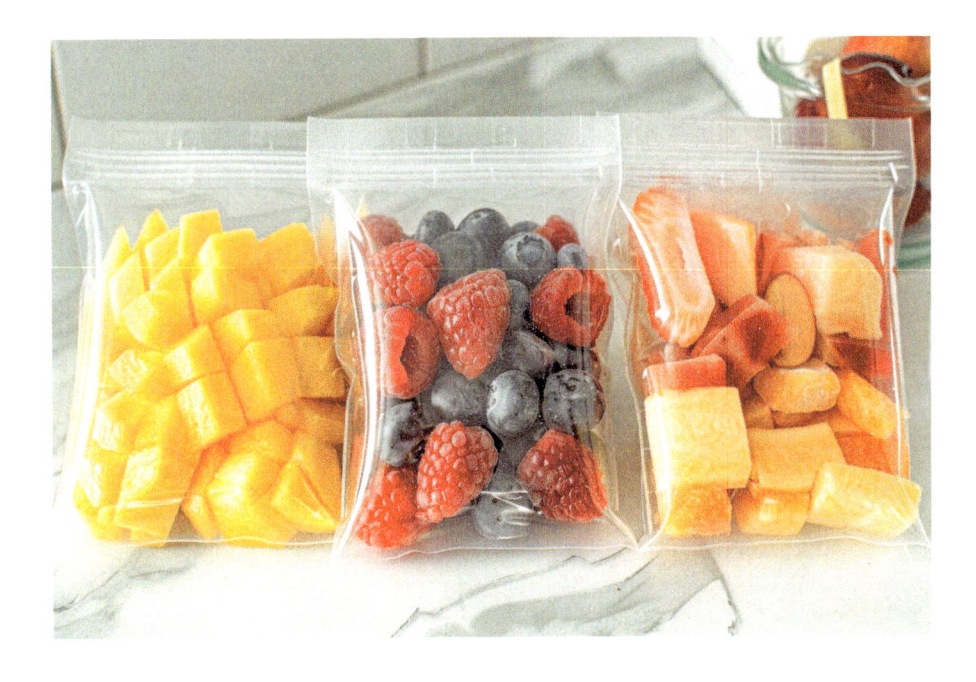

When you've got your hands on beautiful seasonal produce, adjusting your recipes to incorporate these items can bring a refreshing twist to your meals. It's all about flexibility and creativity. Let's say you have a favorite soup recipe that calls for zucchini, but it's not zucchini season—no problem! Try substituting it with another seasonal vegetable like squash or carrots. Keeping your meals exciting and varied allows you to experiment with new flavors and textures while maximizing their nutritional benefits. This adaptability in the kitchen is vital to keeping your anti-inflammatory diet practical and exciting.

Preserving these seasonal flavors can extend the benefits throughout the year. Freezing, canning, and pickling are excellent methods for keeping the bounty of peak seasons. Freezing is one of the easiest techniques, and it works wonderfully for berries, peaches, and even greens like spinach and kale. Just wash, dry, and freeze on a tray before transferring to a freezer-safe bag—this keeps them from clumping together.

Canning is a bit more involved, but it can be a fun weekend project. Imagine making your tomato sauce with vine-ripped tomatoes at their peak or peach preserves from the juiciest, sun-warmed peaches.

Then there's pickling, which extends the shelf life of foods like cucumbers and beets and adds a flavorful zing to meals. Plus, foods prepared these ways retain much of their nutritional value, so you're not just preserving any food—you're keeping good, wholesome nourishment.

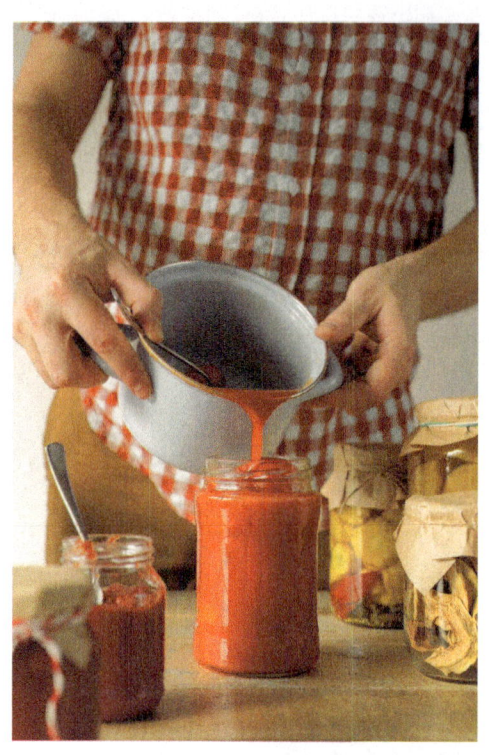

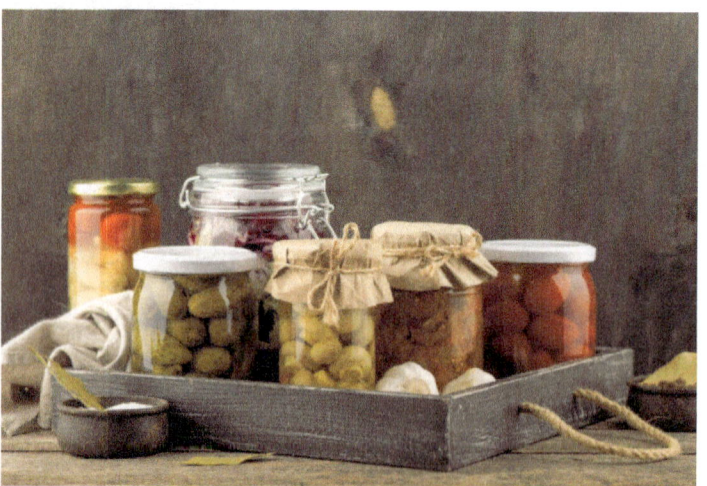

By embracing the rhythm of the seasons, you align your diet more closely with nature's cycles, which can lead to a deeper connection to the food you eat and the world around you. This connection can make eating a more mindful and gratifying experience, enhancing your overall enjoyment and satisfaction with your meals. So, next time you eat a crisp apple in the fall or savor a sweet berry in the summer, take a moment to appreciate the natural cycle that brought that food to your table. It's a beautiful way to nourish both your body and your soul.

ADVANCED MEAL PLANNING: PREPPING FOR SUCCESS

Advanced meal planning can be your best ally in maintaining an anti-inflammatory lifestyle. Think of it as your roadmap through the sometimes overwhelming healthy eating landscape. By planning, you can ensure that your meals meet your nutritional needs and fit seamlessly into your personal preferences and busy schedule. One effective strategy is to develop a rotating meal plan by creating a menu cycle that repeats every few weeks.

The beauty of this system is that it allows you to cater to your dietary needs while also providing variety, which is crucial to keeping your meals exciting and enjoyable. Start by mapping out a week or two of meals that align with your anti-inflammatory goals, then rotate these menus throughout the month. This approach not only saves you from the boredom of eating the same things repeatedly but also simplifies grocery shopping and cooking, as you'll become familiar with the recipes and ingredients.

Now, let's talk grocery shopping. It's easy to get off track when faced with countless food options, many of which might not align with your health goals. To keep your shopping trips efficient and your cart filled with nutrient-rich foods, always go with a list—and stick to it! But here's the kicker: before you even write down what you need, spend a few minutes planning your meals for the week and knowing precisely what to buy, saving time and reducing food waste. In the store, shop the perimeter where fresh produce, meats, and dairy are usually located. The inner aisles tend to house the more processed foods, which you want to limit. Also, consider shopping when stores are less crowded, such as on weekday mornings or late evenings. This can make your shopping experience quicker and less stressful, helping you stay focused on making healthy choices.

Regularly incorporating new recipes into your meal plan is another key to maintaining excitement and commitment to your diet. It's easy to fall into a rut, making the same dishes because they're familiar and easy. However, trying new recipes breaks the monotony and encourages you to eat a wider variety of anti-inflammatory foods, which can enhance your overall nutrient intake. Aim to try one new recipe weekly or swap seasonal ingredients to revamp old favorites. This approach broadens your culinary skills, introduces new textures and flavors, and keeps your diet appealing and nutritionally diverse.

Lastly, let's not overlook the importance of batch cooking and freezing, especially during those ultra-busy periods. Dedicate a few hours each week to prepare and cook large quantities of meals that store well, like soups, stews, casseroles, and marinated proteins. Divide these into meal-sized portions and freeze them. This way, you always have a stock of ready-to-go meals that support your anti-inflammatory diet, saving you from reaching for less healthy alternatives when you're short on time or energy. Make sure to label your containers with the date and contents to keep track of what you have, and use older items first. This method ensures that you have healthy meals on hand when needed and helps manage portion control, which can be crucial for maintaining weight and reducing inflammation.

By mastering these advanced meal planning and prepping techniques, you'll find that eating an anti-inflammatory diet becomes more than just a series of daily decisions—it becomes a sustainable, enjoyable part of your lifestyle. This way, you ensure that every meal nourishes your body, supports your health goals, and brings you joy—no matter how busy life gets.

WHEN TO REASSESS YOUR DIET AND MAKE TWEAKS

Understanding when and how to adjust your diet can be as crucial as the diet itself. Think of it this way: Your life and your body's needs aren't static. Over time, things change—energy levels, health conditions, even your activity levels—and your diet should evolve. Recognizing the signs suggesting it's time to tweak your eating habits can make a significant difference in maintaining optimal health and ensuring your diet meets your needs.

One of the first indicators that it might be time to reassess your diet is a change in your energy levels. Suppose you start feeling unusually tired and sluggish or need to be more sharp mentally. In that case, it might signal that your body isn't getting the right balance of nutrients it needs to function efficiently due to a variety of reasons, such as needing more calories for your specific energy needs, needing more vitamins or minerals, or not getting the right mix of macronutrients. Similarly, changes in digestive health, such as increased bloating, gas, or changes in your bowel habits, can indicate that something in your diet isn't sitting well with your gut. You may have developed a sensitivity to a food you were previously OK with or need more of a particular nutrient to help support digestive health.

Another sign to watch for is the persistence or escalation of inflammation symptoms. If you're primarily following an anti-inflammatory diet to manage a health condition like arthritis, and you notice that your symptoms are flaring up more frequently or intensely, it could be a cue that your current dietary choices need reevaluation. This might mean you need to cut back on certain foods that have crept back into your diet, or it might be an indication to introduce other foods that could help manage inflammation more effectively.

Regular health check-ups are invaluable in this journey. These appointments allow healthcare providers to review the effectiveness of your diet from a medical perspective. Blood tests can reveal much about how your diet affects your health, showing deficiencies or excesses in various nutrients and giving insight into inflammatory markers and other health indicators. These check-ups can lead to adjustments in your diet based on professional medical advice, ensuring that your eating habits continue to support your overall health optimally.

Adapting your diet to life changes is another aspect of dietary reassessment. Our nutritional needs can change dramatically at different stages of life—during pregnancy, while breastfeeding, as we age, or when dealing with a health condition. Each stage may require more or less certain nutrients, and understanding these needs can help you make informed dietary choices. For instance, older adults may need more calcium, vitamin D, and B12, while someone recovering from surgery might need more protein and vitamin C to help repair tissues and heal.

Finally, learning to listen to your body's signals is perhaps one of the most intuitive ways to know when to make dietary changes. Your body can tell you what it needs; sometimes, it's just a matter of tuning in and being receptive. If certain foods make you feel unwell, your body might tell you to cut back on them. Conversely, you might find that you feel more vibrant and energetic when you eat more of certain foods, like those rich in omega-3 fatty acids or antioxidants. Paying attention to these signals can guide you to fine-tune your diet in a way that feels right for you, enhancing your health and well-being in a personalized way.

Adjusting your diet isn't about striving for perfection or adhering rigidly to a set of rules. It's about making responsive changes that align with your evolving health needs and life circumstances. By staying attuned to the signs your body and life are showing you and being proactive about seeking professional health advice, you can ensure that your diet remains a supportive pillar for your health, no matter what changes come your way.

CONTINUING EDUCATION: STAYING INFORMED ON NUTRITIONAL ADVANCES

In the ever-evolving world of nutrition science, keeping your knowledge fresh and up to date is not just beneficial—it's essential. Staying informed about discoveries and perspectives in anti-inflammatory diets can empower you to make the best choices for your health. Think of it as equipping yourself with the latest tools in your wellness toolkit. Learning deepens your understanding and keeps you inspired and committed to your health journey. Let's explore practical ways to stay on top of the latest nutritional science and anti-inflammatory lifestyles.

One of the most dynamic ways to keep learning is by following recent studies and publications. The field of nutrition is bustling with new research, and staying connected to this flow of information can provide valuable insights into how foods affect inflammation and overall health. But where do you start? Academic journals, reputable health websites, and even newsletters from trusted institutions can be gold mines of information. Additionally, books that delve into the science behind anti-inflammatory diets can be both informative and transformative. Consider setting a goal to read one new article or study each week or join a book club focusing on health and wellness topics. This approach keeps you informed and makes learning an enjoyable part of your routine.

Technology also plays a pivotal role in making learning about nutrition more accessible. Numerous apps and online courses offer structured learning right at your fingertips. These resources often provide interactive content like videos, quizzes, and forums where you can discuss topics with other learners. Apps can serve as daily reminders of your learning goals and help track your progress, making education a regular part of your daily life. Look for apps that offer credible, science-backed information and customizable learning paths. Whether you're interested in deepening your understanding of biochemical pathways or simply looking for practical tips on meal planning, there's likely a digital resource that fits your needs.

Networking with professionals specializing in nutrition and anti-inflammatory lifestyles can also significantly enhance your educational journey. Consider scheduling consultations with dietitians or attending talks and seminars they host. These professionals can provide personalized advice tailored to your specific health conditions and dietary needs. Moreover, building a relationship with a healthcare provider who understands the principles of anti-inflammatory eating can be incredibly beneficial.

They can help interpret scientific information, debunk diet myths, and offer guidance based on the latest research, ensuring that the advice you follow is current and clinically sound.

Lastly, community involvement can be a powerful way to reinforce your learning. Joining or forming groups focused on healthy eating and anti-inflammatory lifestyles offers mutual support and motivation. These communities can be found in local health clubs, online platforms, or even among friends and family. Being part of a community allows you to share recipes, cooking tips, and personal experiences, which can enrich your understanding and application of anti-inflammatory principles in real life. It also connects you with individuals who are similarly committed to maintaining their health, providing a network of support that encourages persistence and resilience in your dietary choices.

By embracing these avenues for continuous education, you ensure that your approach to managing inflammation through diet remains informed, effective, and responsive to the latest scientific findings. This commitment to learning enhances your health and equips you to share valuable knowledge with others, spreading the benefits of informed, health-conscious living.

As we wrap up this exploration of ongoing education and its critical role in sustaining an anti-inflammatory lifestyle, remember that knowledge is one of the most potent tools at your disposal. By staying informed, leveraging technology, connecting with experts, and engaging with a community, you continue to build a foundation of understanding that supports your health goals. This proactive approach to learning empowers you to navigate your health journey with confidence and curiosity, ensuring that your dietary and lifestyle choices are always guided by the most current and comprehensive information available. Use this chapter as a stepping stone for further exploration and more profound understanding as you discover and implement the most effective strategies for maintaining a vibrant, healthy life.

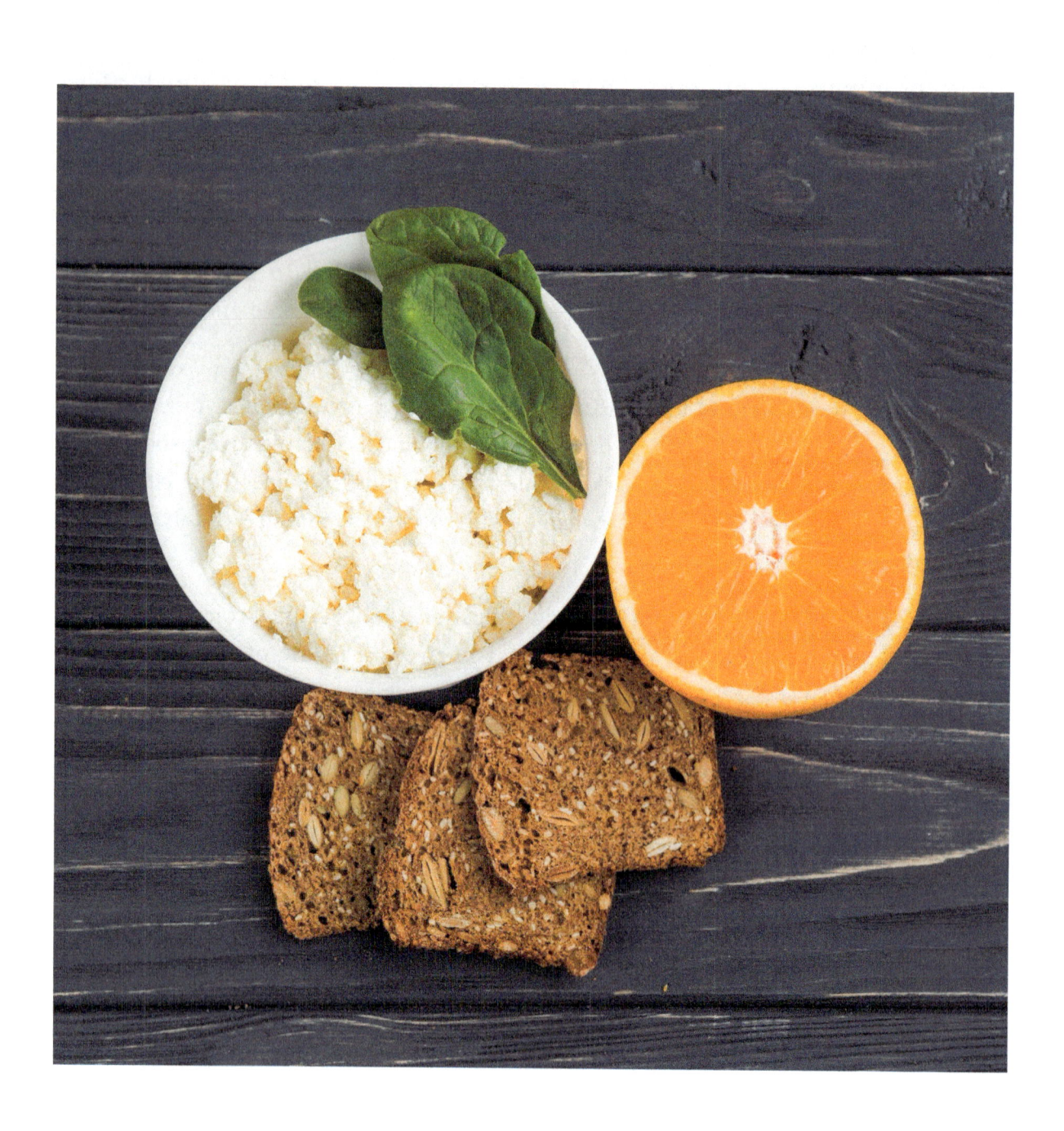

8

QUICK AND EASY ANTI-INFLAMMATORY RECIPES

Starting your day with the proper breakfast sets the tone for the rest of your day. Think of it as laying down the first bricks of a foundation that will support everything you build on it throughout the day. These recipes are quick, straightforward, and packed with nutrients to fight inflammation and energize you until lunch. Whether you're an early riser ready to spend a little time in the kitchen or someone who grabs the first thing you see in the morning, there's something here for you.

FIVE-INGREDIENT BREAKFASTS TO KICKSTART YOUR DAY

Imagine waking up to a breakfast that's not only mouthwatering but also aligns beautifully with your anti-inflammatory goals –and all with just five key ingredients! I developed these recipes to simplify your morning routine while ensuring you start each day packed with nutrition. Let's dive into some of these breakfast ideas:

Oatmeal with Mixed Berries and Cinnamon

Oatmeal is a fantastic breakfast choice due to its high fiber content, which helps reduce inflammation and keeps you feeling full longer. For a delightful twist, mix in fresh or frozen berries—like blueberries, strawberries, or raspberries—for a dose of antioxidants that combat inflammation. A sprinkle of cinnamon not only adds flavor but also offers anti-inflammatory benefits. Here's a tip: Prepare your oatmeal the night before in a jar, layering oats, cinnamon, and berries. Add milk or hot water in the morning, shake it well, and let it sit while you get ready. It's delicious, nutritious, and effortless.

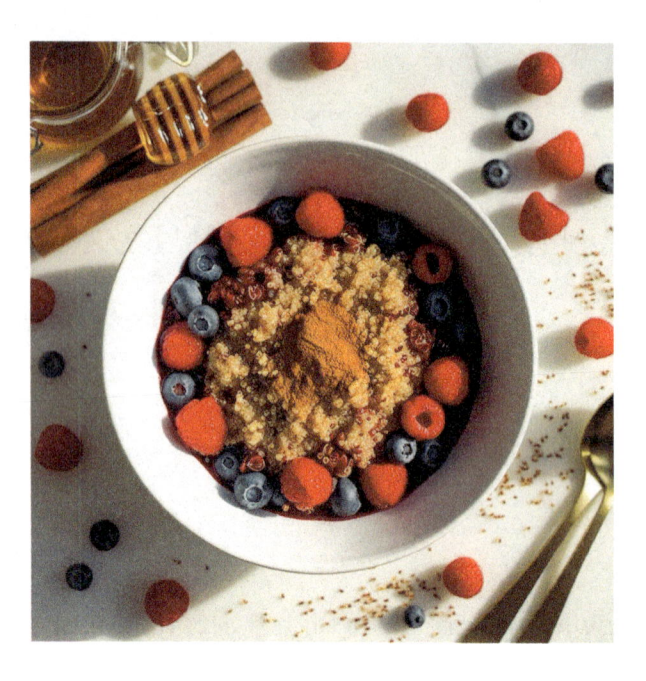

Avocado Toast with Olive Oil Drizzle

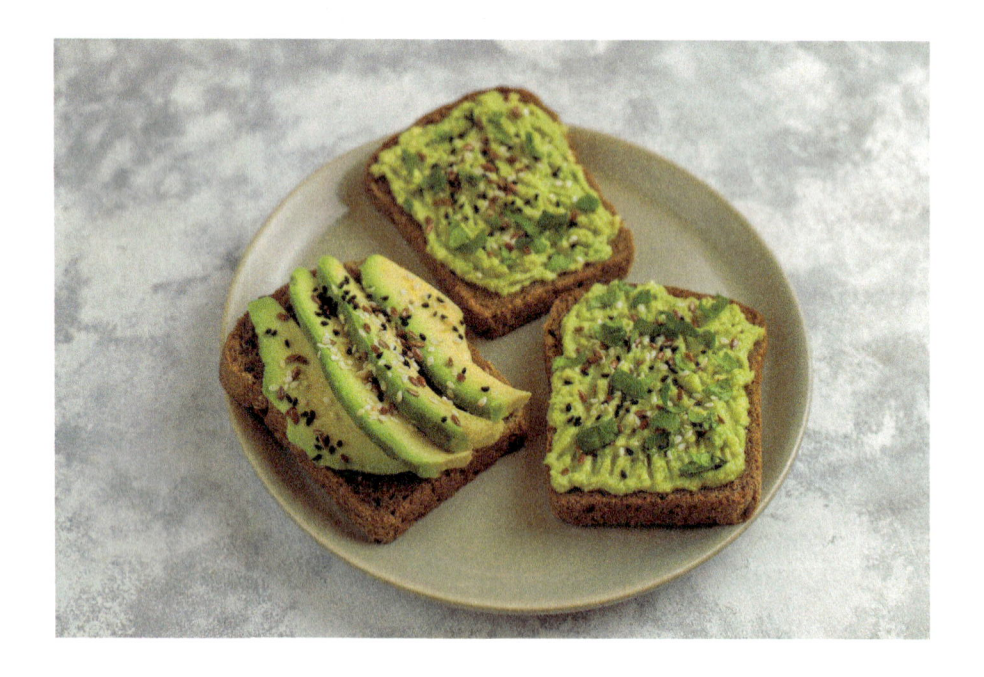

For good reason, avocado toast has become a favorite for breakfast. Monounsaturated fats, abundant in avocados, are excellent for reducing inflammation and supporting heart health. Smash a ripe avocado on a slice of whole-grain toast (gluten-free, if you prefer) and drizzle with olive oil for an added anti-inflammatory boost. Not only does olive oil improve flavor, but it also aids in the absorption of nutrients. For a morning time-saver, slice or smash your avocado the night before, sprinkle it with lemon juice to prevent browning, and store it in an airtight container in the fridge.

Spinach and Mushroom Omelet

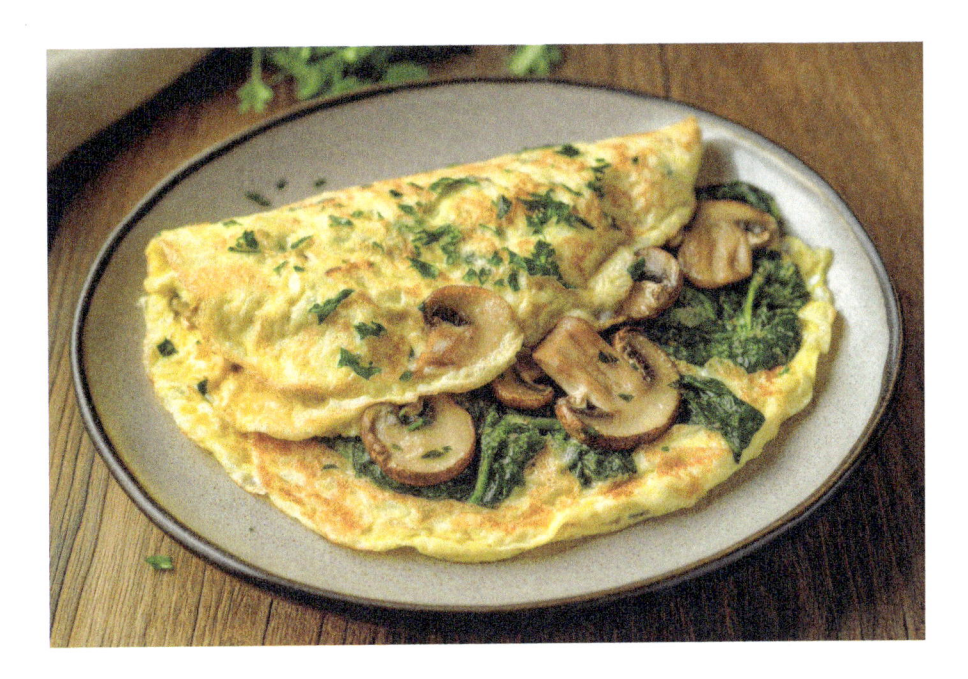

In addition to being exceptionally versatile, eggs are a great source of superior protein. After whisking several eggs, add them to a hot, well-oiled skillet. Add some fresh spinach and sliced mushrooms—the spinach provides an excellent source of vitamins, and mushrooms are known for their anti-inflammatory properties. If you're avoiding dairy, skip the cheese or choose a sprinkle of nutritional yeast or vegan cheese for a flavor boost. To make your morning routine faster, chop the spinach and mushrooms the evening before and keep them in your fridge. It's as simple as morning sautéing, pouring, and cooking.

Balancing macronutrients is vital to these breakfast options. Each recipe includes a good balance of proteins, fats, and carbohydrates, ensuring you start your day with sustained energy and without the spikes and crashes often caused by less-balanced meals. This balance supports your physical activities throughout the morning and helps manage blood sugar levels, which is crucial in controlling inflammation.

Each of these breakfast ideas is flexible for those with specific dietary needs. Using gluten-free oats, dairy-free milk, or egg substitutes can make these dishes suitable for various dietary restrictions without compromising taste or nutritional benefits. The simplicity of these recipes also means you can easily swap one ingredient for another based on availability or preference, making it less of a recipe and more of a template for your creative breakfast creations.

Starting your day with any of these meals nourishes your body and aligns with your anti-inflammatory goals, keeping you on track from when you wake up. Plus, the simplicity and quick prep time means you will maintain healthy eating practices, even on your busiest mornings.

QUICK LUNCHES: MEALS IN 20 MINUTES OR LESS

Lunchtime is that midday break when you pause, relax, and refuel your body to tackle the rest of the day. Who has the time to cook an elaborate meal between work, errands, and a quick gym session? Mastering a few quick, nutritious, anti-inflammatory lunch recipes can make a difference. They say necessity is the mother of invention, and it's true when creating swift and healthy lunches.

One of my favorite go-to methods for a speedy lunch is using a single pan to cook protein and a selection of vegetables, simplifying the cooking process and reducing the amount of washing up. Imagine tossing some chopped chicken breast, bell peppers, zucchini, and onions into a pan and drizzling them with olive oil, salt, pepper, and maybe paprika or turmeric for an anti-inflammatory boost. Sauté everything together until the chicken is cooked thoroughly and the veggies are tender. It's colorful, delicious, and can be prepared in less than 20 minutes. Plus, the combination of lean protein and fibrous vegetables fills you up and provides a sustained release of energy.

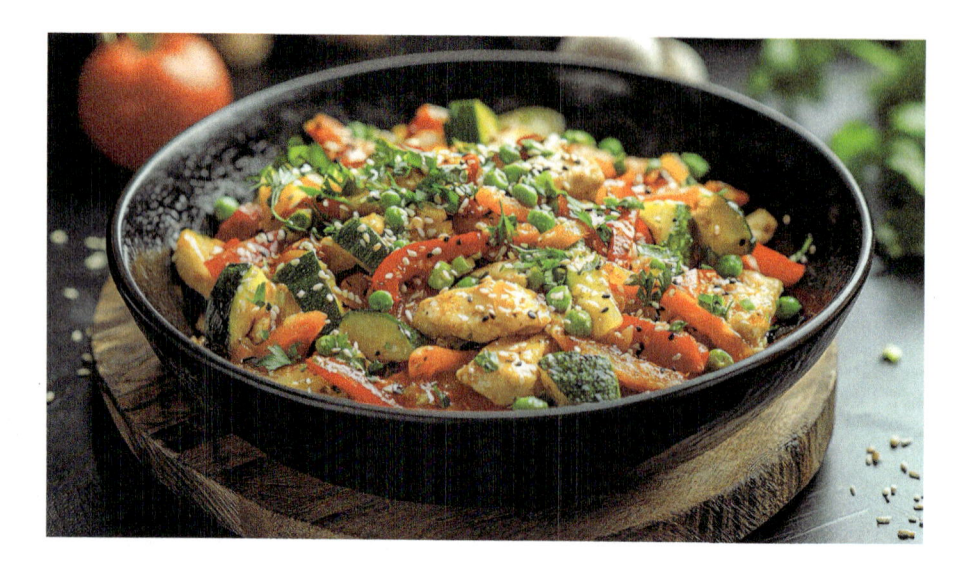

QUICK AND EASY ANTI-INFLAMMATORY RECIPES | 111

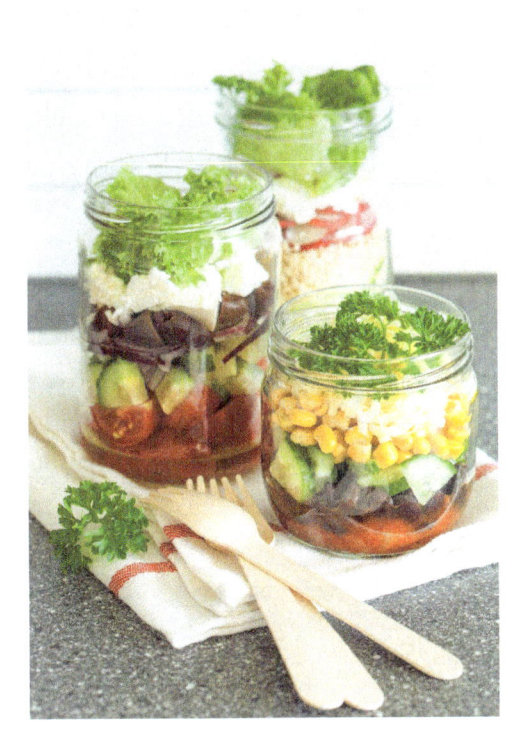

For those days when you're running out the door and need something portable, mason jar salads or wraps are lifesavers. Here's a quick layering idea for a mason jar salad: Start with a dressing base—an essential combination of lemon juice and olive oil. Then, add harder vegetables like carrots or cucumbers, followed by beans or grains for protein. Finally, top with leafy greens like spinach or arugula. When you're ready to eat, shake up the jar and mix your salad, ready to enjoy.

Wraps are equally convenient. Spread some hummus on a whole grain or gluten-free tortilla, layer on some mixed greens, slices of turkey, or a handful of chickpeas, add some sliced avocado for healthy fats, roll it up, and you're good to go. These options are quick to prepare and infinitely customizable based on what you have in your fridge.

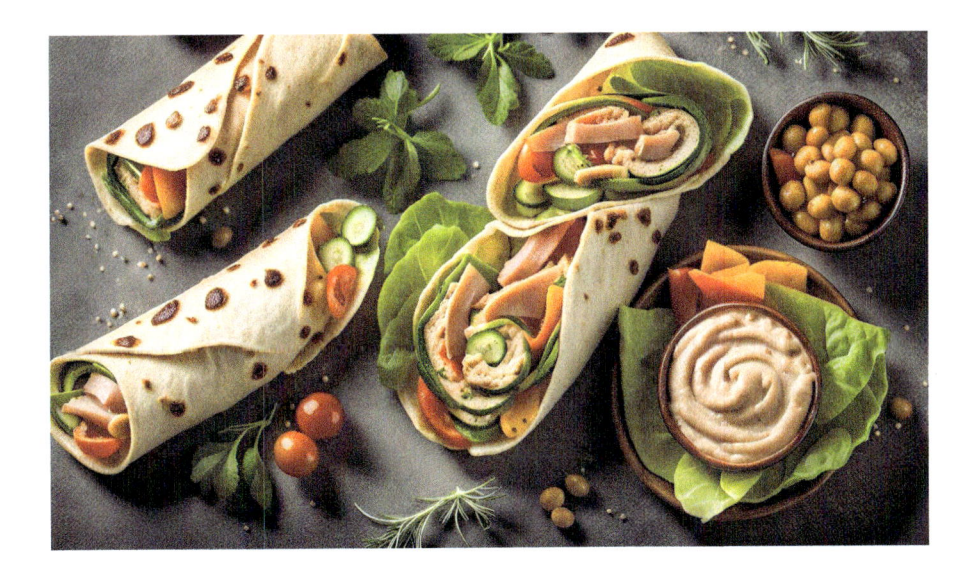

Now, let's talk about one of the most innovative ways to manage time and resources: using leftovers. Transforming last night's dinner into today's lunch is an efficient and economical way to ensure you stick to your anti-inflammatory eating plan without extra cooking. That quinoa and vegetable stir-fry from dinner? Toss it into a skillet, crack an egg over it, and get a new meal with little effort. Or take the leftover roasted chicken, shred it, and add it to a soup with fresh vegetables and herbs. It's about getting creative, seeing the potential in the foods you already have, cutting down on food waste, and simplifying your meal prep significantly.

Remember what you're drinking while focusing on your solid foods. Staying well-hydrated is crucial and another opportunity to keep inflammation at bay. Sipping on herbal teas like ginger or turmeric may be immensely calming throughout the day.

And beneficial due to their anti-inflammatory properties. If you prefer cold drinks, infusing water with slices of cucumber, lemon, or mint makes hydrating more enjoyable. These additions can also aid digestion and further reduce inflammation. Always having a bottle of this infused water or a thermal cup of herbal tea on hand means you're more likely to keep sipping throughout the day, keeping hydration levels optimal.

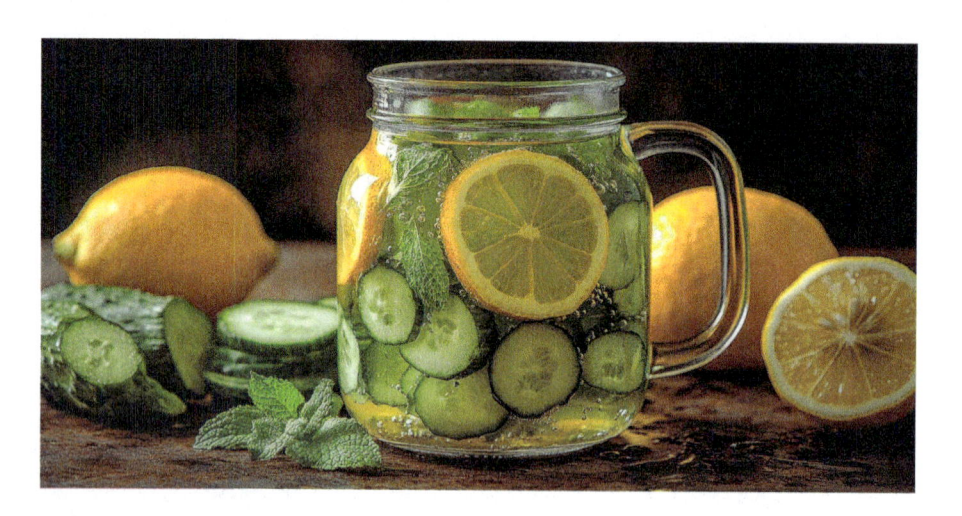

These lunch ideas are designed to be flexible, quick, and aligned with your anti-inflammatory goals. They require minimal prep time, can be altered based on your palate and available resources, and support your health without compromising flavor or satisfaction. Whether you're cooking at home or packing something to take along, these ideas ensure that your midday meal is something to look forward to, supplying your body with energy and satisfying your palate without requiring much time or effort.

SIMPLE AND SATISFYING ANTI-INFLAMMATORY DINNERS

Dinner is more than just a meal; it's a chance to unwind from the day's hustle, nourish your body, and spend quality time with loved ones. Crafting dinners that align with your anti-inflammatory goals can be straightforward. Embracing techniques like batch cooking will streamline your meal preparation and ensure delicious, healthy options are readily available throughout the week. Let's explore how you can transform your dinner routine into an efficient yet enjoyable part of your day.

One of the best strategies for simplifying your dinner routine is to embrace the concept of batch cooking. This approach involves preparing large quantities of versatile dishes to serve in various ways over several meals. Think hearty vegetable stews rich in anti-inflammatory spices like turmeric and ginger or a big casserole dish filled with layers of roasted vegetables, lean proteins, and whole grains.

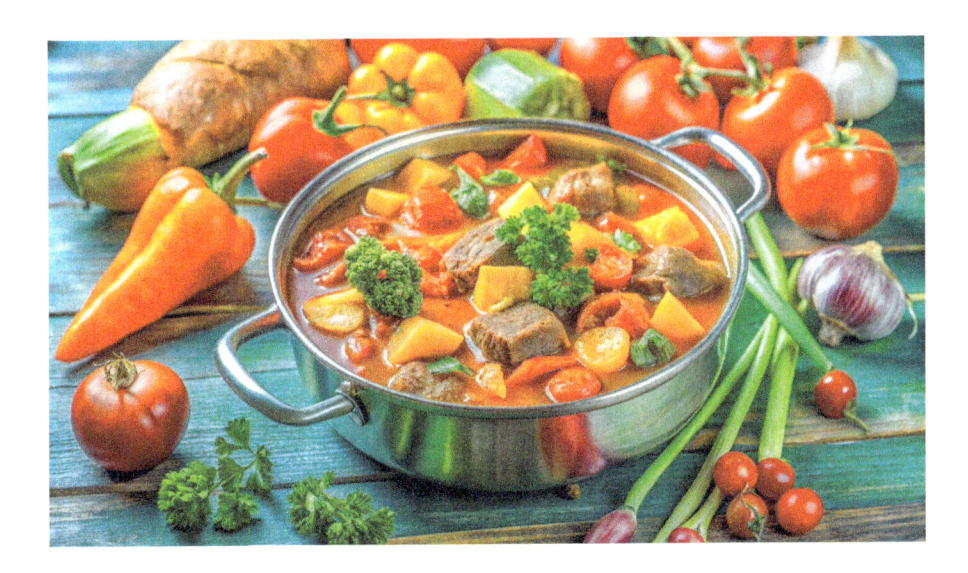

These dishes usually taste even better the next day as the flavors have more time to meld together. They can easily be reheated, saving time and energy on busy evenings. Another great option is to prepare a large pot of soup. Soups are incredibly forgiving and versatile, allowing you to toss in various ingredients—like leafy greens, beans, and root vegetables—that you need to use. They're perfect for simmering on a lazy Sunday afternoon and can provide comforting meals throughout the week.

If you're short on time but still want a dinner that supports your anti-inflammatory diet, you can prepare plenty of dishes in about 30 minutes. A simple yet flavorful option is to stir-fry various vibrant veggies, including broccoli, bell peppers, and snap peas, paired with your preferred protein source, such as tofu or chicken. Use garlic, ginger, and a splash of low-sodium soy sauce or tamari for a quick, delicious sauce. Another fast and nutritious dinner option involves baking a salmon fillet seasoned with herbs and lemon, served alongside a quinoa salad tossed with sliced cucumber, cherry tomatoes, and a drizzle of olive oil.

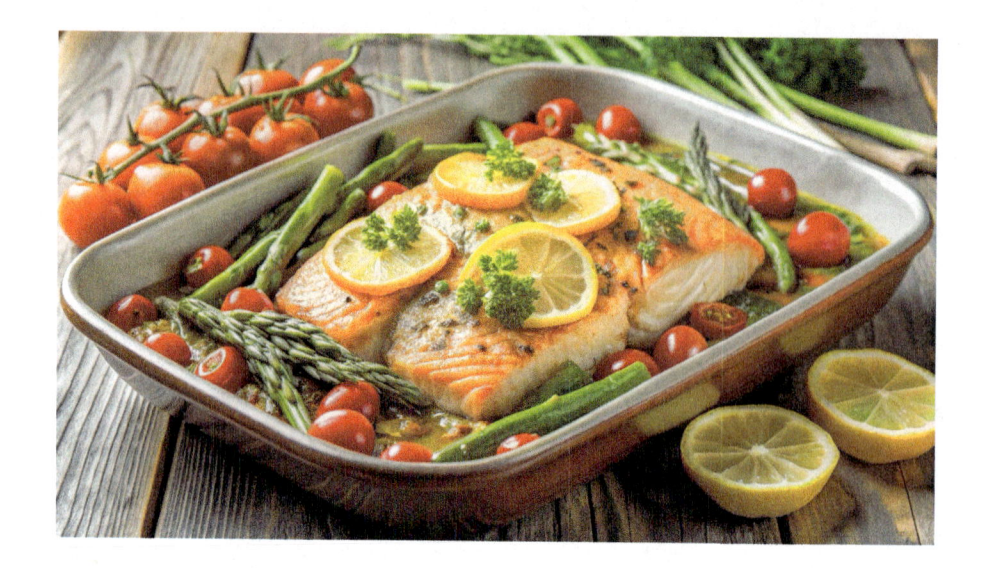

These meals are quickly prepared and packed with the nutrients needed to fight inflammation and boost your overall health.

Including your family in the cooking process can be an excellent way to spend time together and encourage healthy eating habits. Kids can help with tasks like tearing up leafy greens, stirring mixtures, or setting the table, and they're more likely to be interested in the meal if they've had a hand in preparing it. Cooking together also allows you to teach them about the benefits of eating whole, nutrient-rich foods and how these foods help keep our bodies strong and healthy. Plus, it's fun to have everyone working together in the kitchen, and it can turn meal preparation from a chore into an enjoyable family activity.

Lastly, focusing on seasonal and locally sourced ingredients can significantly enhance your meals' flavor and nutritional value. Seasonal produce is typically fresher and more flavorful, which can make a big difference in your cooking. Visit your local farmers' market to see what's in season, and don't be afraid to try new ingredients. Not only are you likely to stumble upon some delicious new favorites, but you're also lessening the environmental effect of long-distance food transportation and helping regional farmers.

You can keep your meals exciting and diverse by experimenting with flavors and textures using local, fresh foods. By incorporating these strategies—batch cooking for convenience, preparing quick 30-minute meals, involving the family, and using fresh, seasonal ingredients—you can ensure that your dinners are not only straightforward and stress-free but also supportive of your anti-inflammatory lifestyle. Each meal becomes an opportunity not just to eat but to nourish and connect, making dinnertime a highlight of your day.

SNACKS AND SMALL BITES: HEALTHY OPTIONS ON THE GO

Maintaining energy levels is crucial to the rhythm of daily life, and smart snacking plays a pivotal role in this. Snacks are not just treats; they're strategic tools to fuel your body throughout the day, ensuring you don't hit a midmorning slump or an afternoon crash. Snacking wisely on an anti-inflammatory diet can help you maintain your energy levels without causing your blood sugar to increase. Foods that release energy slowly—think fiber-rich fruits, nuts, and yogurt—keep you feeling fuller longer and your blood sugar stable. This keeps you alert and curbs those cravings that might have you reaching for something less healthy.

Preparing snacks in advance is a game-changer. It takes the guesswork out of what you can eat, especially when you're busy or on the go. Consider making a batch of roasted chickpeas over the weekend. Just rinse and pat dry the chickpeas, then toss them with olive oil and your favorite spices—maybe a dash of sea salt, paprika, and garlic powder. Roast them in the oven until they're crispy. These make for a crunchy, protein-rich snack that's easy to pack and take with you. Another great option is homemade granola bars.

Mix oats, your choice of nuts and seeds, and maybe some dried fruit for sweetness, and bind them with a bit of honey or maple syrup. Press the mixture into a pan, bake, and then cut into bars. These are healthier than many store-bought options, which can be high in sugar and preservatives but are also customizable to your taste and nutritional needs.

Regarding snacking throughout the day, it's wise to align your snacks with your body's energy needs, which change as the day progresses. In the morning, when you're kick-starting your metabolism, a piece of fruit might be all you need to accompany your breakfast, giving you a quick burst of energy. In the afternoon, when you might need a more substantial boost to get through the rest of the day, something like a small yogurt with a handful of nuts or a slice of whole-grain toast with almond butter offers a perfect mix of proteins, fats, and carbohydrates. In the evening, a lighter snack like raw veggies and hummus or a small salad can tide you over until dinner without feeling too heavy.

Let's make snacking interactive and fun, especially if you have kids or enjoy a bit of variety. Creating a "build-your-own" trail mix station at home can be a delightful way to customize your snacks.

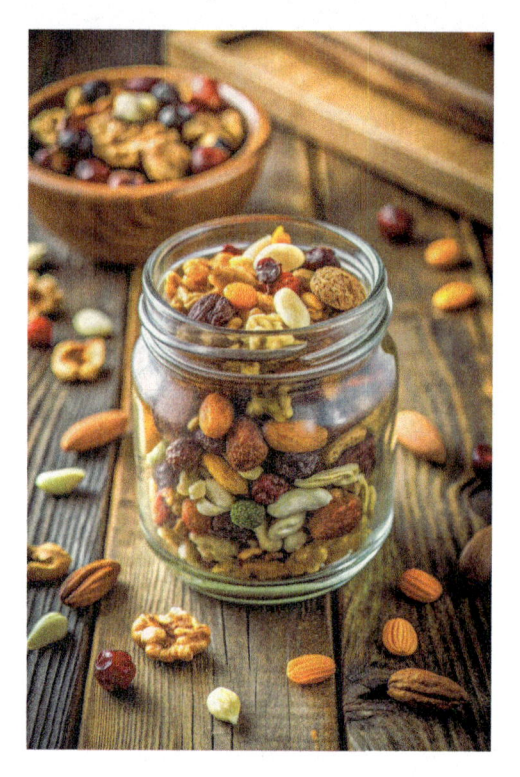

Set out jars of different ingredients, like various unsalted nuts, seeds (pumpkin, sunflower, chia), dried fruits (cranberries, apricots, coconut strips), and maybe some dark chocolate chips for a touch of sweetness. Anyone can combine different items to match their taste and dietary needs, making unique trail mix combinations. Personalizing your snacking ensures you know the ingredients, helping you avoid unwanted sugars, salts, or oils commonly found in pre-packaged products.

Embracing these snacking habits transforms the act from a mere eat-to-satisfy-craving to a thoughtful way to fuel your body, keeping your energy levels stable and your mind focused. Preparing these healthy snacks ensures you're always ready with a quick bite that's not only delicious but also keeps you aligned with your anti-inflammatory goals, no matter where your day takes you. Whether you're at home, at work, or on the move, these snack ideas provide the perfect balance of convenience and nutrition, making healthy eating seamless and enjoyable every day.

DELICIOUS SMOOTHIES, JUICES, DRINKS, AND HERBAL TEAS FOR INFLAMMATION RELIEF

Smoothies, juices, and herbal teas are not just refreshing; they pack a substantial nutritional punch that can significantly impact your anti-inflammatory efforts. Imagine starting your day or refreshing yourself after a workout with a drink that cools you down and fills you with antioxidants, vitamins, and minerals. By integrating superfoods like berries, turmeric, and flaxseeds into these beverages, you can turn them into powerful allies against inflammation.

Smoothies and Juices: Blending and Juicing for Maximum Benefits

Superfoods are not just a trendy term; they bring profound benefits to the table—or, in this case, the blender. With their high levels of antioxidants, berries aid in lowering oxidative stress, a significant cause of inflammation in the body. Turmeric, a bright yellow spice, contains curcumin, which is known for its potent anti-inflammatory properties. Omega-3 fatty acids, abundant in flaxseeds, have been shown to reduce inflammation. Combining these ingredients into a smoothie isn't just about flavor; it's about creating a concentrated, delicious dose of anti-inflammatory agents.

For instance, blending a handful of mixed berries, one teaspoon of turmeric (with a sprinkle of black pepper to improve absorption), a tablespoon of ground flaxseeds, some Greek yogurt, and a splash of almond milk can yield a potent anti-inflammatory beverage that's both delicious and nutritious.

Understanding the distinctions between blending and juicing is crucial for optimal results. Blending involves mixing whole fruits and vegetables, keeping the fiber intact. Fiber aids digestion, slows blood sugar absorption, and helps you feel full, which can be beneficial for weight management. On the other hand, juicing extracts the liquid from fruits and vegetables, removing most of the fiber and delivering a more concentrated form of vitamins and minerals. While you miss out on fiber, you get a more easily digestible shot of nutrients, which can be beneficial for those with sensitive stomachs or those looking to give their digestive system a light day.

Each method has its place in an anti-inflammatory diet, and alternating between them can provide various health benefits. For instance, a morning juice made from celery, cucumber, a small amount of ginger, and green apple can be a refreshing way to hydrate and invigorate your body without feeling too full—perfect for those mornings when you're not quite ready for a heavy breakfast. A blended smoothie, meanwhile, is excellent for a post-workout meal or a substantial snack to fuel your afternoon activities.

Variety is the spice of life, which also holds true for your smoothies and juices. Everyone's taste preferences and nutritional needs are different, so here are a few recipes to cater to a range of palates:

The Green Booster: Blend spinach, a small green apple, half a banana, a handful of parsley, a teaspoon of chia seeds, and a squeeze of lemon juice. This drink is packed with iron, potassium, and protein, making it a tremendous, energizing start to your day.

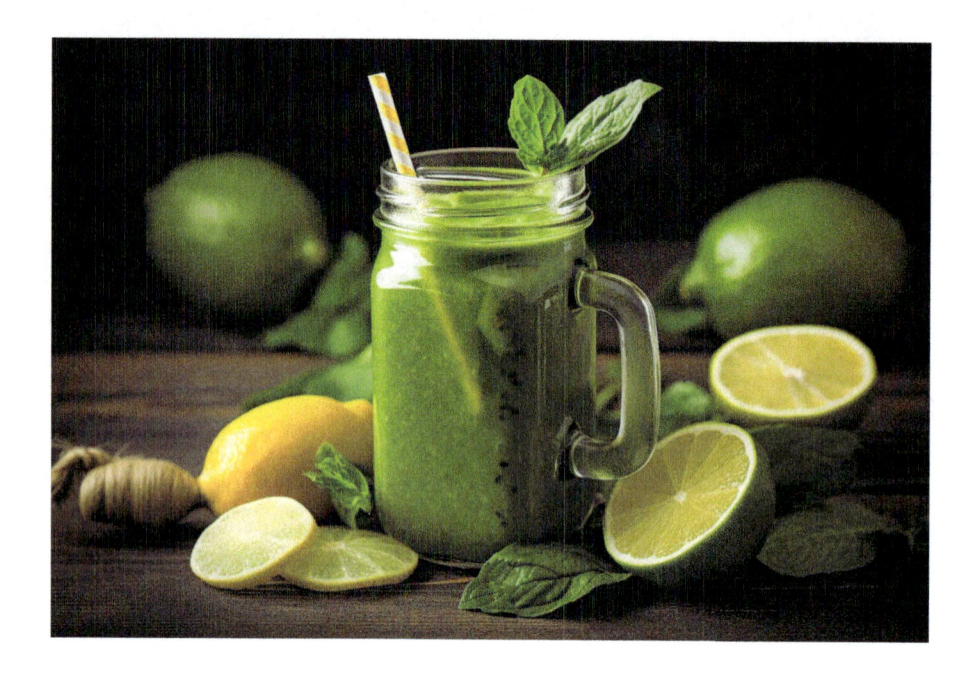

The Berry Anti-Inflammatory: Juice a cup of mixed berries, a small beet, a carrot, and a small piece of peeled turmeric root. This juice is stunningly vibrant and loaded with antioxidants and anti-inflammatory compounds.

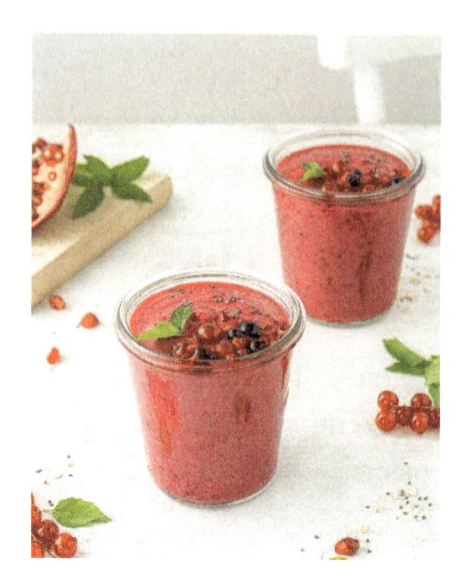

The Tropical Turmeric Smoothie: Blend a cup of pineapple chunks, half a banana, a tablespoon of coconut oil, a cup of coconut water, and a teaspoon of turmeric. This smoothie is tropical, hydrating, and anti-inflammatory—perfect for a post-sunshine cool-down.

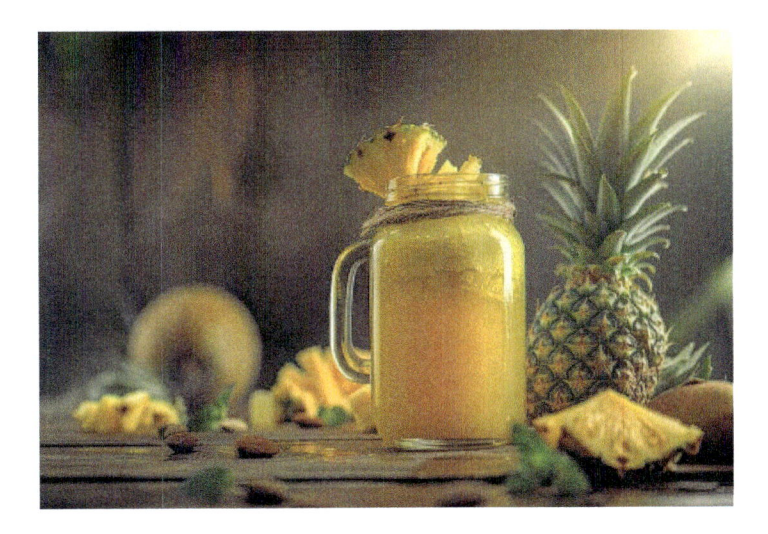

Incorporating these smoothies and juices into your morning routine can be a delightful and refreshing way to start your day. You can save time in the morning by preparing everything the night before, making this healthy habit fit seamlessly into your busy schedule. Imagine opening your fridge to find all your ingredients ready to go, transforming your morning rush into a moment of creative, nutritious tranquility. Whether you choose a smoothie or a juice, each sip is a step toward a more energized, less inflamed you, making every glass a treat and a vital part of your health regimen.

Herbal Teas for Inflammation Relief

In addition to smoothies and juices, herbal teas offer another simple yet powerful way to support your body's natural defense against inflammation. These teas have been cherished for centuries for their comfort, warmth, and health benefits. Certain herbal teas are particularly known for their anti-inflammatory properties due to their rich content of phytochemicals—natural compounds that work to reduce inflammation and boost overall well-being.

Green Tea: Rich in polyphenols, particularly catechins like EGCG, green tea is a potent anti-inflammatory. These compounds help reduce inflammation at the cellular level and have been shown to lower the risk of chronic diseases such as heart disease and cancer.

Chamomile: Known for its calming effects, chamomile also contains flavonoids like apigenin, which have anti-inflammatory and antioxidant properties. Drinking chamomile tea can help reduce gastrointestinal inflammation and improve sleep quality, further aiding in the reduction of overall inflammation.

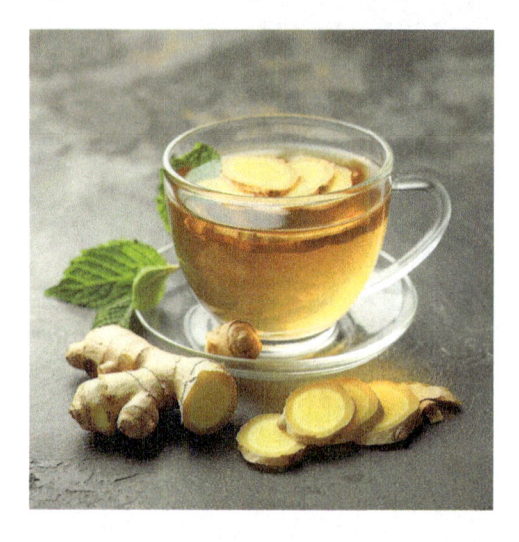

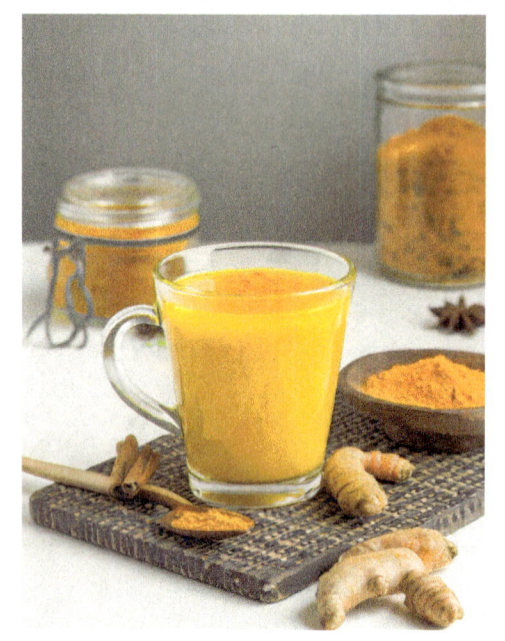

Ginger: Ginger tea is made from the root of the ginger plant and is loaded with gingerols and shogaols—powerful compounds that inhibit the production of inflammatory cytokines. It's particularly beneficial for easing joint pain and improving digestive health.

Turmeric: The bright yellow spice that gives curry its color, turmeric is packed with curcumin, a compound with strong anti-inflammatory effects. Turmeric tea, often enhanced with a pinch of black pepper to improve absorption, is a powerful addition to any anti-inflammatory diet.

Peppermint: Peppermint tea contains rosmarinic acid, which has been shown to reduce symptoms of seasonal allergies and soothe the digestive tract. Its cooling effect can also help alleviate headaches and muscle soreness, making it a versatile anti-inflammatory option.

Detoxifying and Speciality Drinks

Detox drinks can be a great way to kickstart your day or refresh your body after a workout. These drinks are not only hydrating but also help to flush out toxins and reduce inflammation.

- **Lemon Water**: Start your day with a glass of warm lemon water. The vitamin C in lemons helps neutralize free radicals in the body, reducing inflammation. Plus, it aids digestion and supports liver function.
- **Turmeric Shots**: Mix 1 teaspoon of turmeric powder with the juice of half a lemon, a pinch of black pepper, and 1 tablespoon of honey in a shot glass of warm water. This potent shot can be taken in the morning to jumpstart your immune system and combat inflammation.
- **Golden Milk (Turmeric Latte)**: Golden milk, also known as turmeric latte, is a soothing and warming drink that combines the anti-inflammatory power of turmeric with the calming properties of warm milk.

Basic Golden Milk Recipe:

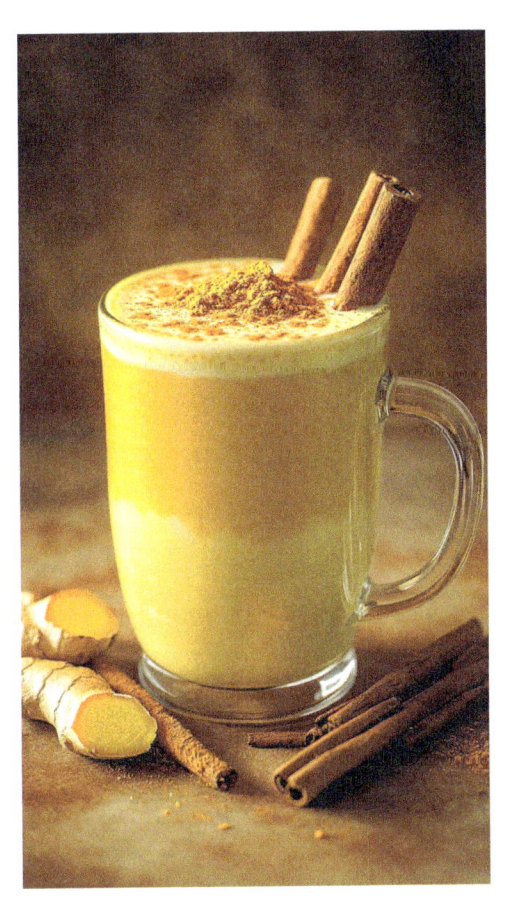

1 cup of your choice of milk (almond, coconut, or dairy)

1 teaspoon turmeric powder

1/2 teaspoon cinnamon

1/4 teaspoon ginger powder

1 tablespoon honey or maple syrup (optional)

A pinch of black pepper

Heat the milk in a small saucepan over medium heat. Whisk in the turmeric, cinnamon, ginger, and black pepper. Sweeten with honey or maple syrup if desired. Serve warm.

Variations: For an extra kick, add a pinch of cayenne pepper or a splash of vanilla extract. You can also blend in a teaspoon of coconut oil for added richness and health benefits.

Daily Beverage Planning for Optimal Inflammation Relief

Incorporating these drinks into your daily routine is easier than you might think. Here's a sample plan:

- **Morning**: Start with a glass of lemon water or a turmeric shot to wake up your digestive system.
- **Midmorning**: Sip on green tea or a ginger smoothie for a midmorning energy boost.
- **Afternoon**: Enjoy a fresh juice like carrot-beet-celery or a cup of chamomile tea to help keep inflammation at bay.
- **Evening**: Wind down with a cup of peppermint tea or a comforting mug of golden milk to relax and reduce inflammation before bed.

Remember to balance these drinks with plenty of water throughout the day to stay hydrated and support your body's natural detoxification processes. By making these anti-inflammatory beverages a regular part of your routine, you'll be well on your way to reducing inflammation and improving your overall health.

DESSERTS: SATISFYING YOUR SWEET TOOTH THE RIGHT WAY

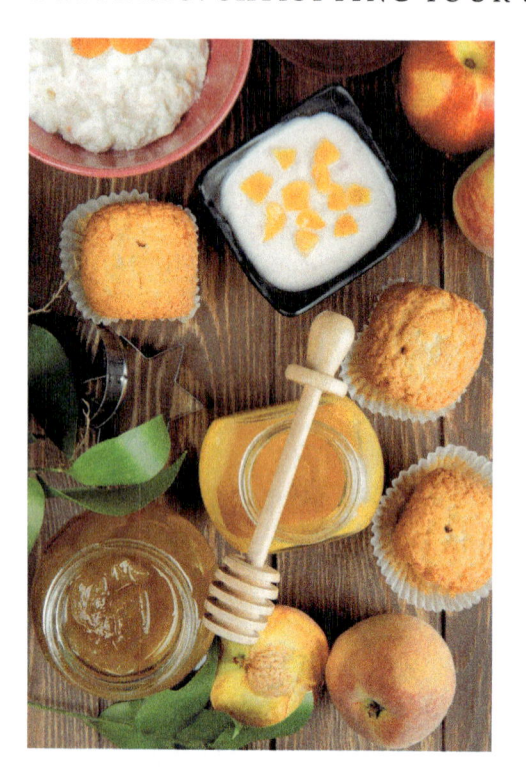

Who says you can't indulge a little while using an anti-inflammatory diet? Let's redefine what dessert means by whipping up some sweet treats that satisfy those sugary cravings and align with your health goals. You can prepare delightful and nourishing desserts by choosing natural sweeteners, incorporating fruits, and integrating healthy fats.

It's important to know that not all sweeteners are created equal, starting with natural sweeteners. Traditional desserts frequently contain refined sugars, raising blood sugar levels and exacerbating inflammation. On the flip side, natural sweeteners like honey, maple syrup, and stevia offer sweetness without the adverse effects of processed sugar. Honey, for instance, sweetens your desserts and contains antioxidants and antibacterial properties. A great alternative is maple syrup, which has essential elements like manganese and zinc that help your body fight off infections. A great choice if you're watching your calorie intake is Stevia, a sugar substitute manufactured from the leaves of the Stevia plant that contains no calories. It's much sweeter than sugar, so a little goes a long way. Incorporating these natural sweeteners into your desserts means you can indulge in a sweet delicacy without being concerned about the inflammation that traditional sugars might cause.

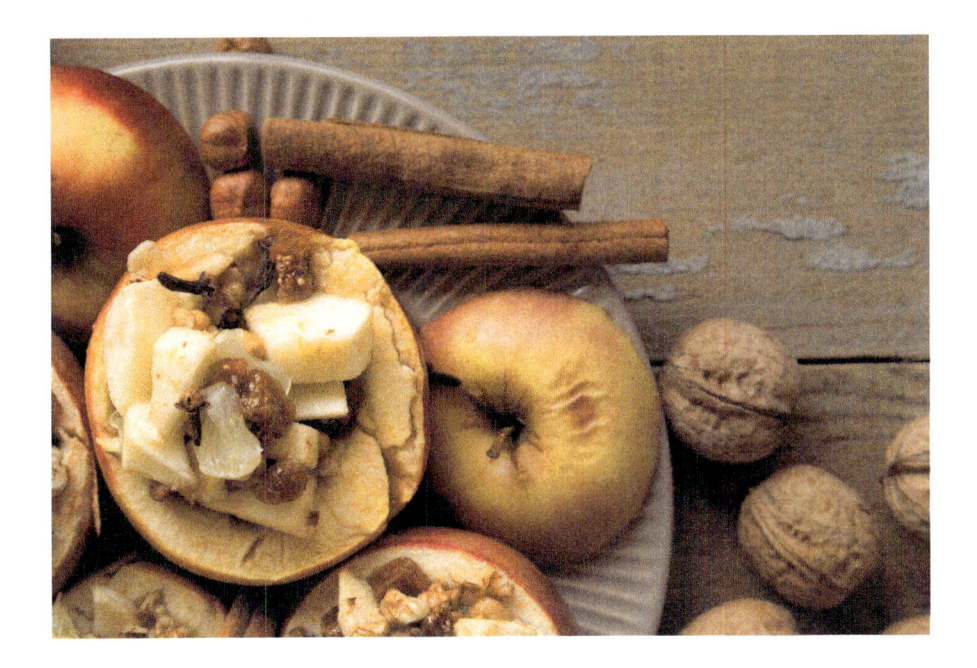

Fruit-based desserts are another excellent way to indulge wisely. Fruits are nature's candies with vitamins, minerals, and fibers that help fight inflammation. An easy and delightful dessert option is baked apples sprinkled with cinnamon and a dash of honey. This simple dish amplifies the natural sweetness of the apples, while cinnamon adds a comforting spice that boosts your metabolic health. Another quick, refreshing option is berry sorbet. Blend frozen berries with a splash of orange juice and a drizzle of honey, then freeze. This satisfies your sweet tooth and infuses your body with antioxidants found in berries, which are great for reducing inflammation.

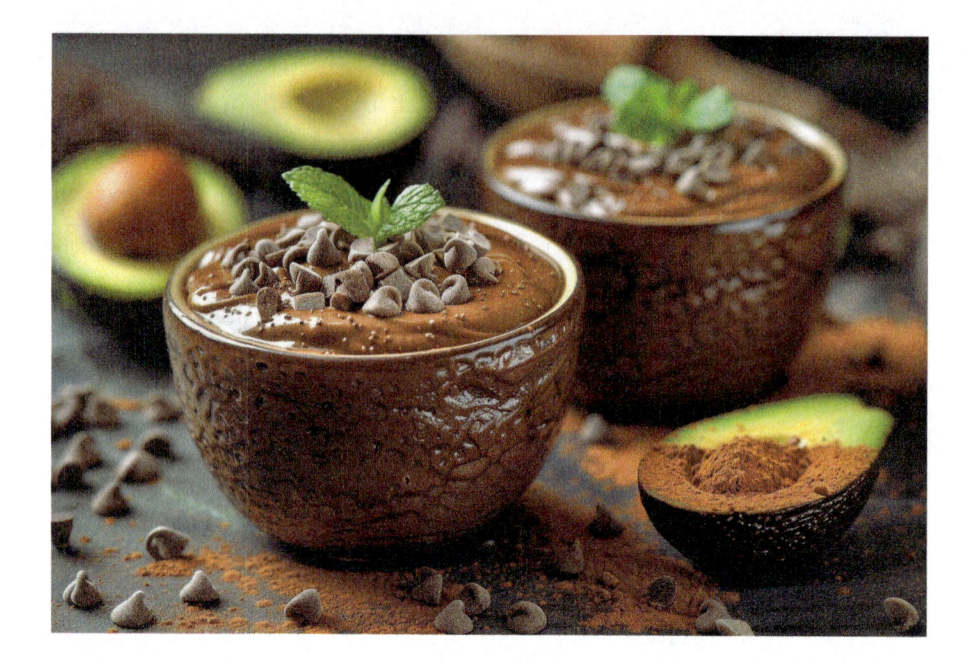

Let's remember the role of healthy fats in desserts. Ingredients like avocados and nuts add a rich texture and contribute essential fatty acids vital for managing inflammation. Avocado chocolate mousse, for example, uses the creamy texture of avocados mixed with cocoa powder and a bit of honey to create a decadent, chocolaty dessert that's completely guilt-free.

Almonds and walnuts can be added to cookies or crumbles, offering a satisfying crunch plus omega-3 fatty acids known for their anti-inflammatory properties.

Lastly, plenty of options fit the bill for those special occasions when you want to whip up something festive yet health-conscious. A fruit tart, with a base of nuts and dates topped with a lush layer of coconut cream and fresh, colorful fruit, can be a show-stopper at any gathering. Not only is it visually appealing, but it's also packed with nutrients and void of the usual inflammatory ingredients found in traditional desserts. Creating these desserts transforms indulgence into nourishment. Each option is easy to make and offers the richness and sweetness you crave.

Through thoughtful ingredient choices and simple preparations, these desserts not only conclude your meals on a sweet note but also contribute to your overall well-being, keeping inflammation at bay.

As we wrap up this tasty chapter on quick and easy anti-inflammatory recipes, remember that each meal and snack provides an opportunity to nourish your body and support your health goals. From the simplicity of five-ingredient breakfasts to the convenience of quick lunches, from the heartiness of satisfying dinners to the sweet indulgence of desserts, each recipe is crafted to enhance your dietary journey without extra stress or time commitment. The focus has been on flavors, simplicity, and nutrition, ensuring you can effortlessly enjoy delicious meals and snacks that support your anti-inflammatory lifestyle.

KEEPING THE GAME ALIVE

Now that you have everything you need to **reduce chronic inflammation, improve gut health, manage weight loss, and enhance immunity**, it's time to pass on your newfound knowledge and show other readers where they can find the same help.

By sharing your experience, you can help someone just like you—someone who is looking for a way to take control of their health and transform their life. Your review might be the beacon of hope that guides them to the answers they've been searching for.

Please take a moment to leave a review.

Your review not only supports the mission to make the anti-inflammatory diet accessible to everyone but also keeps the game alive by empowering others to embark on their journey toward better health.

Simply scan the QR code below to leave your review:

https://www.amazon.com/review/create-review/?asin=B0DQDZYSLZ

Thank you for being a part of this movement.

Together, we're making the world a healthier place—one review at a time.

With gratitude,
Lynn Benedetto

CONCLUSION

As we wrap up our journey through the vibrant and nourishing world of the anti-inflammatory diet, I want to reflect on all that we've covered. From exploring the significant benefits of managing weight loss, improving gut health, reducing inflammation and pain, and boosting immunity, it's clear that what we put on our plates can powerfully influence our health and well-being.

Remember when we started this journey together? We began by unpacking the complexities of inflammation—understanding its roots and how it affects our body. We moved through the essential knowledge needed to adopt an anti-inflammatory lifestyle, from identifying critical foods to embracing whole, natural ingredients. We didn't just talk about what to eat; we made it practical with easy-to-follow recipes and meal plans that simplify the transition to healthier eating.

One of my main goals was to show you that this diet isn't just accessible; it's doable, no matter your starting point. We've broken down the science into bite-sized pieces that are easy to digest and apply. Whether whipping up a quick breakfast or planning a week's worth of meals, I hope you now see that incorporating anti-inflammatory foods into your daily routine can be as simple as beneficial.

If you still need to do so, please take that first step. Embrace the changes, however small, and remember that each meal is an opportunity to nourish and heal your body. It's not about perfection; it's about making better choices one day at a time. Consistency is essential, and patience is a virtue in this journey toward better health.

Let's remember the power of a holistic approach. Combining your diet with regular physical activity and mindfulness can amplify your results, transforming your physical health and mental and emotional well-being. As you grow more accustomed to this lifestyle, keep your curiosity alive. The world of nutritional science is constantly evolving, and staying informed will help you refine and optimize your diet to suit your changing health needs.

No one should have to walk this path alone, so I also encourage you to seek out communities and professionals who can support and guide you. Connecting with others who share your health goals can boost motivation and accountability, whether online or in person.

Finally, I want to leave you with a personal note of encouragement. My passion for helping others achieve their health goals stems from a deep belief that we all deserve to live our most-whole, healthiest lives. You have the power to combat inflammation and enhance your well-being, one meal at a time. Embrace the challenge, trust the process, and remember—I'm cheering for you every step of the way.

Here's to a healthier, more vibrant you!

REFERENCES

Ajmera, Rachael. "8 Gluten-Free Grains That Are Super Healthy." Healthline, September 25, 2019. https://www.healthline.com/nutrition/9-gluten-free-grains.

Alexis, Amber Charles. "What Does the Evidence Say about Anti-Inflammatory Diets?" MedicalNewsToday, March 18, 2022. https://www.medicalnewstoday.com/articles/do-anti-inflammatory-diets-really-work.

Ansley, Hill. "Anti-Inflammatory Diet 101: How to Reduce Inflammation Naturally." Healthline, December 13, 2018. https://www.healthline.com/nutrition/anti-inflammatory-diet-101.

APA. "Mindfulness Meditation: A Research-Proven Way to Reduce Stress," October 30, 2019. https://www.apa.org/topics/mindfulness/meditation.

Ball, Jessica. "The 6 Best Budget-Friendly Anti-Inflammatory Foods, According to a Dietitian." EatingWell, January 15, 2023. https://www.eatingwell.com/article/8024844/best-budget-friendly-anti-inflammatory-foods/.

Bjarnadottir, Adda. "How to Read Food Labels Without Being Tricked." Healthline, February 27, 2019. https://www.healthline.com/nutrition/how-to-read-food-labels.

Bjarnadottir, Adda. "Mindful Eating 101 — A Beginner's Guide." Healthline, June 19, 2019. https://www.healthline.com/nutrition/mindful-eating-guide.

Chacon, Tiffany. "11+ Best Kitchen Tools for EASY Healthy Eating in 2023." *Mommy of Mayhem* (blog), May 5, 2021. https://mommyofmayhem.com/kitchen-tools-for-healthy-eating/.

DeAngelis, Danielle. "20 Anti-Inflammatory Lunches You Can Make in 10 Minutes." EatingWell, July 5, 2024. https://www.eatingwell.com/gallery/7967197/anti-inflammatory-lunches-in-10-minutes/.

Elliot, Catherine Anne, and Michael John Hamlin. "Combined Diet and Physical Activity Is Better than Diet or Physical Activity Alone at Improving Health Outcomes for Patients in New Zealand's Primary Care Intervention." *BMC Public Health* 18, no. 1 (February 8, 2018): 230. https://doi.org/10.1186/s12889-018-5152-z.

Evans, Dillon. "18 Anti-Inflammatory Desserts You'll Want to Make Forever." EatingWell, July 12, 2023. https://www.eatingwell.com/gallery/8057591/anti-inflammatory-desserts-to-make-forever/.

Goggins, Leah. "38 Anti-Inflammatory Dinners You Can Make in 30 Minutes." EatingWell, April 6, 2023. https://www.eatingwell.com/gallery/7946056/anti-inflammatory-dinner-recipes-in-30-minutes/.

Greenfield, Sarah. "5 Must-Read Social Dining Tips for People with Dietary Restrictions." Fearless Fig, Dec 14. https://www.fearlessfig.com/blog/dietary-restrictions-social-dining-tips.

Hanley, Ryan. "The Exact Anti-Inflammatory Diet Meal Plan That Changed My Life." *Ryan Hanley* (blog), December 12, 2018. https://ryanhanley.com/anti-inflammatory-diet-meal-plan/.

Harvard Health Publishing. "Quick-Start Guide to an Anti-inflammation Diet," May 1, 2020. https://www.health.harvard.edu/staying-healthy/quick-start-guide-to-an-antiinflammation-diet.

Harvard Health Publishing. "Stress and The Sensitive Gut," August 1, 2010. https://www.health.harvard.edu/newsletter_article/stress-and-the-sensitive-gut.

Hewings-Martin, Yella. "What Is the Gut Microbiome and Why Is It Vital for Health?" ZOE, n.d. https://zoe.com/learn/the-gut-microbiome-and-your-health.

Hill, Ansley. "23 Tips to Ease Meal Prep." Healthline, July 8, 2019. https://www.healthline.com/nutrition/meal-prep-tips.

Johns Hopkins Medicine. "Anti Inflammatory Diet," February 20, 2024. https://www.hopkinsmedicine.org/health/wellness-and-prevention/anti-inflammatory-diet.

Levy, Sue. "I USED FOOD AS MEDICINE So Can You!" Savory Living, June 13, 2019. https://www.savoryliving.com/my-story-food-as-medicine.

Lutz, Jennifer. "Obesity and Inflammation: A Vicious Cycle." HealthCentral, June 25, 2020. https://www.healthcentral.com/condition/obesity/obesity-inflammation-cycle.

Marengo, Katherine. "What to Eat and Drink to Boost Your Immune System." Healthline, April 30, 2020. https://www.healthline.com/health/food-nutrition/foods-that-boost-the-immune-system.

MariGold Makers. "Gut Health 101: Top Prebiotic and Probiotic Foods." *MariGold Foods* (blog), September 9, 2020. https://www.marigoldfoods.com/gut-health-101-top-prebiotic-and-probiotic-foods/.

Mount Sinai Health System. "Low FODMAP Diet: Understanding FODMAPs," n.d. https://www.mountsinai.org/health-library/selfcare-instructions/low-fodmap-diet.

Petr, Alina and Ajmera, Rachael. "The 18 Best Protein Sources for Vegans and Vegetarians." Healthline, August 16, 2016. https://www.healthline.com/nutrition/protein-for-vegans-vegetarians.

Schulte, Sadie. "24 Anti-Inflammatory Breakfasts with 5 Ingredients or Less." Yahoo Life, April 24, 2024. https://www.yahoo.com/lifestyle/24-anti-inflammatory-breakfasts-5-200304194.html.

Six, Hannah. "Chronic Inflammation: Why It's Harmful, and How to Prevent It." Novant Health | Healthy Headlines, August 11, 2023. https://www.novanthealth.org/healthy-headlines/chronic-inflammation-why-its-harmful-and-how-to-prevent-it.

Tambe, Dr. Rahul. "Maintain a Healthy Life? Here's a Importance of Regular Health Check-Ups." Nanavati Max, August 11, 2023. https://www.nanavatimaxhospital.org/blogs/importance-of-regular-health-check-ups.

U.S. Food & Drug Administration. "Milk and Plant-Based Milk Alternatives: Know the Nutrient Difference," n.d. https://www.fda.gov/consumers/consumer-updates/milk-and-plant-based-milk-alternatives-know-nutrient-difference.

Wartenberg, Lisa. "The 13 Most Anti-Inflammatory Foods You Can Eat." Healthline, December 20, 2019. https://www.healthline.com/nutrition/13-anti-inflammatory-foods.

Wolf's Apple House. "Modifying Recipes to Cook with the Seasons," August 3, 2016. https://wolffsapplehouse.com:443/modifying-recipes/.

Zając, Aleksandra and Mucha, Mateusz. "Harris-Benedict Calculator (Basal Metabolic Rate)." OMNI Calculator, June 7, 2024. https://www.omnicalculator.com/health/bmr-harris-benedict-equation.